LOW IMPACT EXERCISE FOR WOMEN

Beginners step by step guide for weight Loss, Enhanced Flexibility, balance, joint relief and improved Core Strength 7 minutes daily

Shelby L. Becker

TABLE OF CONTENT

INTRODUCTION — 5

Chapter 1: Getting Started — 9

  Assessing Your Fitness Level — 13

  Setting Realistic Goals — 18

  Planning Your Workout Routine — 22

Chapter 2: Why Low-Impact Exercise Matters — 27

  Benefits for Women's Health — 31

  Joint-Friendly Workouts — 35

  Boosting Confidence and Energy — 41

Chapter 3: Strength and Tone — 46

  Using Resistance Bands — 50

  Bodyweight Exercises — 54

  Pilates and Barre Workouts — 59

Chapter 4: Aquatic Exercise — 64

  Water's Therapeutic Benefits — 69

  Water Aerobics — 73

  Swimming for Fitness — 78

Chapter 5: Walking for Wellness — 83

  Walking Techniques — 87

  Interval Walking — 91

  Enjoyable Walking Routes — 95

Chapter 6: Balance and Stability   **99**
    Balance Exercises   103
    Core Strength Training   107
    Yoga and Tai Chi   111
Chapter 7: Relaxation and Stress Relief   **115**
    Meditation Techniques   119
    Relaxation Practices   123
    Deep Breathing Exercises   127
CONCLUSION   **131**

INTRODUCTION

Tessy resided in Willow Creek, a pleasant suburban area surrounded by colorful fall colors. Tessy was a loyal wife, a compassionate mother, and a hardworking employee.

Her days were filled with the obligations of her family and profession, leaving little time for self-care. Tessy's physical and emotional obligations became increasingly burdensome over the years.

Despite her best attempts to manage her responsibilities, Tessy began to feel the effects of her sedentary lifestyle. Aches and aches infiltrated her body, settling in her neck and back like unwanted visitors. Joint pain became a daily companion, a reminder of the years of neglect her body had suffered.

Simple chores like stooping down to tie her shoes or lugging groceries were difficult obstacles.

The stress of everyday life further increased Tessy's physical suffering. Every day it seemed like a marathon with no end in sight. Her obligations pushed down on her like a big stone, threatening to crush her spirit under them. Tessy yearned for comfort, a break from the constant anguish that haunted her every waking hour.

Tessy discovered a glimpse of hope on one especially rough afternoon. One day, she came across low-impact Exercise for Women, the exercise tool she needed that emphasized the benefits of gentle movement and attentive breathing.

With nothing to lose and everything to gain, Tessy decided to give it a go. She created a small area in her living room and began moving her body in ways she hadn't done in years. At first, it was difficult; her muscles resisted the new exercise, and her breath came in short, ragged gasps. But, gently and surely, Tessy felt the tension dissipate.

Tessy continued day after day, steadfastly committed to low-impact exercise. With each session, she felt stronger, more resilient, and more alive. Her neck and back pains faded, and she felt lighter and more at peace. Joint discomfort faded into memory, a relic of a period when she neglected herself.

Tessy, encouraged by her renewed vigor, decided to share her story with those closest to her. She introduced her sisters to the benefits of low-impact exercise, supporting them on their journey to self-discovery and regeneration. They laughed, sweated, and cheered each other on, forming ties as strong as steel and as soft as morning dew.

As the seasons changed and the years passed, Tessy remained strong in her determination to live life to the fullest. She relished the basic joys of movement and attentiveness, taking every breath as if it were her last. Though she was aware of the obstacles that remained ahead, she embraced them with bravery and elegance, certain that she had recaptured her best self - body, mind, and soul.

Chapter 1: Getting Started

Beginning a fitness journey may be both thrilling and intimidating, especially when considering low-impact workouts. These workouts are mild on the joints yet provide major health advantages.

Incorporating low-impact activities into women's routines can improve cardiovascular health, muscle strength, weight management, and general well-being. Here's a complete guide on getting started.

1. Consult with a Healthcare expert: Before starting any fitness program, speak with a healthcare expert, especially if you have any pre-existing medical ailments or concerns.

2. Set Realistic Goals: Decide what you want to achieve with your low-impact workout program. Setting reasonable and achievable objectives, whether they are for increasing flexibility, enhancing cardiovascular health, or weight management, will help you stay motivated.

3. Select Appropriate Activities: Low-impact workouts include walking, swimming, cycling, yoga, Pilates, and tai chi. Choose activities that you love and that are consistent with your fitness objectives.

4. Begin Slowly: Begin with short, 10-15-minute workouts, gradually increasing the time and intensity as your fitness improves. To avoid injury, maintain good form and technique.

5. Warm-Up and Cool Down: Always begin with a mild warm-up that prepares your muscles and joints for activity.

torso twists, arm circles and leg swings are dynamic Stretches that can be included

Similarly, complete each practice with a cooldown to reduce muscle pain and increase flexibility.

6. *Listen to Your Body:* Pay attention to how you feel during and after exercise. If you are experiencing pain or discomfort, alter your activities or take a rest. It's critical to push yourself to your limits without overexertion.

7. *Incorporate Strength Training:* Women require strength training to maintain muscular mass, bone density, and metabolic health. Include workouts that target key muscle groups using body weight, resistance bands, or modest weights.

8. *Stay Hydrated and Fuel Your Body:* Stay hydrated by drinking lots of water before, during, and after your workout. Fuel your body with nutritional nutrients that offer energy and aid in muscle rehabilitation.

9. *Monitor Your Progress:* Keep track of your progress by logging your exercises, taking measurements, or utilizing fitness apps. Celebrate your accomplishments along the road to keep motivated.

10. *Be Consistent:* Consistency is essential for seeing outcomes. Aim for at least 150 minutes of moderate-intensity activity per week, distributed across many days.

Starting a low-impact workout program for women involves careful preparation, focus, and patience. By following these steps and listening to your body, you may get the many advantages of physical exercise while reducing your chance of injury.

Assessing Your Fitness Level

Understanding where you stand is critical in your fitness journey. As a woman, embracing low-impact workouts adds a particular depth to your fitness path, focusing on joint health and general well-being. Here's a unique guide designed to help you measure your fitness level and include low-impact activities into your regimen.

Begin by performing a tailored fitness assessment based on your specific requirements and goals. Evaluate aspects such as cardiovascular endurance, muscular strength, flexibility, and balance.

Tailor evaluations to your interests, such as measuring your progress with mindful walks, bodyweight workouts, or flexibility routines.

Empower yourself by making unique, achievable objectives that are in line with your desires. Setting specific goals, whether they be to enhance heart health, muscular tone, or flexibility, gives a road map for your fitness journey and drives motivation.

Embrace the Mild Approach: Recognize the mild but effective nature of low-impact activities designed for women.

Explore a wide range of activities, including moderate yoga flows, water exercises, cycling, tai chi, and resistance band workouts. These workouts benefit your body while minimizing joint stress, making them suitable for women of all ages and fitness levels.

Mindful Progression: Work at your speed and include mindful progression into your exercise program. Begin with basic motions, emphasizing good form and technique. Increase the intensity and duration of your exercises as you gain strength, stamina, and confidence.

Develop a comprehensive approach to body mechanics to maximize the advantages of low-impact workouts. Throughout each action, pay attention to your alignment, posture, and breathing strategies. Develop body awareness to avoid injury and maximize the efficacy of your workouts.

Strength from inside: Use the power of strength training to shape and strengthen your body from the inside. Use bodyweight exercises, resistance bands, or small weights to target main muscle groups. Muscle strengthening not only improves athletic performance but also benefits bone health and metabolic efficiency.

Celebrate Self-Care and Self-Compassion: Accept self-care and compassion as essential components of your fitness path. Listen to your body's indications and respect its demands. If you become uncomfortable throughout your workout, reduce the intensity or try different activities. Cultivate a loving mentality that values health and well-being over perfection.

By taking this unique method to analyze your fitness level and adding low-impact workouts designed specifically for women, you will go on a journey of self-discovery and empowerment. Celebrate the beauty of movement, respect your body's wisdom, and flourish in your quest for holistic health.

Setting Realistic Goals

Setting realistic objectives is essential for success in any activity, especially when including low-impact activities in a woman's fitness regimen.

Low-impact workouts are mild on the joints, making them appropriate for women of all ages and fitness abilities. To guarantee long-term adherence and growth, set objectives that are both reasonable and attainable.

First and foremost, while defining goals for low-impact workouts, individual fitness levels and restrictions must be considered.

Every woman is unique, and what is tough for one may be too simple or strenuous for another. Begin by examining your current fitness level, as well as any ailments or conditions that may be interfering with your workout performance.

Next, establish clear and quantifiable goals. Rather than attempting to "get in shape," set realistic goals such as increasing flexibility, boosting cardiovascular endurance, or toning specific muscle regions.

A practical aim may be to do 30 minutes of low-impact exercise, such as walking or swimming, three times each week.

It is also critical to establish realistic deadlines for accomplishing these objectives. While it is normal to expect fast results, long-term growth requires patience.

Be patient and realistic about the duration required to complete each milestone. Setting short-term, attainable objectives might help you stay motivated and avoid frustration.

Consider adding diversity to your low-impact training regimen to avoid boredom and plateaus. This might include attempting new hobbies like yoga, Pilates, cycling, or water aerobics. Setting objectives for exploring new things or perfecting certain methods may make exercises more interesting and pleasant.

In addition to physical goals, remember to consider mental well-being. Setting aside time for relaxation and stress management is equally vital as physical activity. Consider integrating meditation, deep breathing exercises, or mild stretching into your daily routine to enhance overall well-being.

Accountability may also play an important part in goal attainment. Whether you seek the aid of a buddy or hire a personal trainer, having someone to hold you responsible may boost motivation and keep you on track.

Finally, enjoy your accomplishments along the road, no matter how minor. Recognizing improvement, whether it's greater flexibility, endurance, or just adhering to a training routine, may enhance confidence and promote good habits.

Setting realistic objectives is critical for success when combining low-impact activities into a woman's fitness regimen.

Women can develop a comprehensive and sustainable approach to fitness that promotes overall health and well-being by taking into account individual limitations, setting specific goals, establishing achievable timelines, incorporating variety, prioritizing mental well-being, seeking accountability, and celebrating progress.

Planning Your Workout Routine

Building a fitness regimen is more than just following a template; it's about creating a path that meets your requirements and interests. For women who prefer the delicacy of low-impact activities, this is an opportunity to develop a complete regimen that honors uniqueness while improving overall well-being.

1. Accept Your Fitness Narrative.
Start by acknowledging your narrative and goals. Your fitness path is as individual as you are, influenced by your experiences, difficulties, and goals. Embrace this story as you create a fitness regimen that represents your beliefs and aspirations.

2. *Foster Collaboration:* Consultation is more than just requesting opinions; it also promotes collaboration. Collaborate with fitness professionals, coaches, or supportive communities to develop a plan that

recognizes your body's strengths and limits while pushing you to progress.

3. *Create a Movement Palette:* Exercise is an art form, and your body is the canvas. Create a palette of low-impact exercises that speak to your spirit. Explore the fluidity of swimming, the elegance of yoga, the rhythm of cycling, or the calm of Pilates, and combine them to create a symphony of wellbeing.

4. *Balance cardio and strength training* : for optimal fitness. Combine aerobic activities such as dancing or hiking with strength training regimens including resistance bands or bodyweight exercises. Allow each note to blend, creating a symphony of life and strength.

5. *Plan Your Workout Routine:* Workouts require both time and dedication. Choreograph your calendar with precision, carving out time for movement within life's pace. Incorporate meaning and purpose into every step, whether it's a dawn yoga session or an evening stroll.

6. *Listen to Your Body's Melody:* Your body communicates through whispers and echoes. As you work your way through each exercise, pay close attention to the music. Honor its cues by modifying tempo and intensity to match its beat, resulting in a symphony of harmony and wellness.

7. *Improve Flexibility and Balance:* Graceful movement requires flexibility and balance. Stretches, balancing postures, and mindful movement techniques such as Tai Chi can all help to elevate these aspects. Allow each stretch and sway to develop a sense of poise and balance inside.

8. *Compose Your Wellness Sonata:* Your fitness path is a continuous symphony of self-discovery and development. Compose it with purpose and passion, connecting the dots of activity, nutrition, and self-care to create a masterpiece of energy and joy.

9. *Pause to ponder, refine, and delight throughout your journey's crescendo:*

Celebrate each accomplishment, learn from each failure, and perfect your routine with wisdom and grace. Accept the symphony of development and progress with open arms.

10. *Dance with Abandon:* Make your fitness journey joyful and liberating. Let go of your inhibitions, accept spontaneity, and move with enthusiasm. For in the rhythm of movement is the melody of life's most authentic expression.

With this unique method of designing your fitness journey, which incorporates the beauty and gentleness of low-impact workouts, you may begin on a road of self-discovery and well-being that aligns with your soul's innermost wishes. Make your trip a symphony of vigor, elegance, and empowerment.

Chapter 2: Why Low-Impact Exercise Matters

Low-impact workouts are essential for women's fitness regimens since they provide several benefits such as less chance of injury, increased joint health, and improved general well-being.

These workouts provide a milder alternative to high-impact activities, making them ideal for women of all ages and fitness levels.

Whether you're recuperating from an accident, managing chronic diseases, or simply searching for a safer method to keep active, including low-impact workouts in your routine is critical for preserving good health and longevity.

Low-impact exercise is important for women since it reduces the chance of injury. High-impact exercises, such as jogging or plyometrics, can put tremendous pressure on the joints, resulting in strains, sprains, and even fractures, particularly in women who are more prone to specific musculoskeletal conditions.

Women may engage in physical activity without putting their bodies under too much strain by choosing low-impact exercises such as swimming, cycling, or walking, which reduces the probability of overuse injuries and promotes long-term joint health.

Low-impact workouts are especially good for women who have pre-existing joint issues or are recuperating from an injury. High-impact sports can be especially difficult for those with osteoarthritis or osteoporosis, potentially exacerbating their symptoms.

Women can successfully manage these illnesses while experiencing the benefits of regular physical activity by opting for low-impact workouts that provide moderate motions with minimum joint stress. Individuals undergoing therapy for injuries can also employ low-impact workouts to develop strength and mobility while avoiding additional injury.

Another compelling reason to favor low-impact exercise is its beneficial effect on overall health. Physical activity is essential for mental health since it helps to reduce stress, anxiety, and sadness.

Women, who sometimes juggle various duties and experience specific challenges, might benefit greatly from regular exercise.

Low-impact workouts offer a long-term strategy to improve mood and energy levels, allowing women to receive the mental health advantages of physical activity without feeling overwhelmed or weary.

Low-Impact workouts are versatile and accessible, making them appropriate for women of different ages and levels of fitness. These exercises, whether conducted at home, at a gym or outdoors, are simply adaptable to meet the needs and preferences of each individual.

Women have a wide choice of alternatives to select from, including mild yoga sessions and low-intensity aerobics courses, ensuring that they can choose activities that match their interests and skills.

Low-impact exercise is an essential component of women's fitness routines, since it provides both physical and mental health advantages.

Women may lower their risk of injury, manage chronic diseases, and improve their general well-being by emphasizing joint-friendly activities. Low-impact exercise, with its variety and accessibility, offers women a long-term approach to being active and healthy.

Benefits for Women's Health

In today's fast-paced world, prioritizing health and wellbeing is critical, especially for women who frequently balance several tasks and obligations.

Incorporating low-impact activities into their daily routines may be transformative, providing several physical, mental, and emotional advantages. Let's look at the overall benefits of low-impact exercise for women's health.

1. Joint Health: Low-impact workouts like swimming, cycling, and walking provide moderate movement that lowers joint stress, making them suitable for women of all ages, especially those who suffer from joint pain or arthritis. These activities enhance flexibility and mobility without putting too much load on the joints, hence improving joint health over time.

2. _Cardiovascular Fitness:_ Low-impact cardiovascular exercise improves circulation, lowers blood pressure, and reduces the risk of heart disease and stroke. Brisk walking or utilizing an elliptical machine increases heart rate without putting the body under high-impact stress, making them safe and effective alternatives for women looking for cardiovascular advantages.

3. _Weight Management:_ Low-impact activities can help women maintain or decrease weight. While they may not burn calories as quickly as high-impact sports, they do contribute to calorie expenditure and metabolic rate, which aids in weight management when paired with a healthy diet.

4. *Stress Reduction:* Regular low-impact exercise increases the production of endorphins, neurotransmitters that reduce stress and improve mood.

Whether doing yoga, tai chi, or moderate stretching exercises, these activities allow women to decompress, de-stress, and improve their overall feeling of well-being.

5. *Bone Density:* Osteoporosis, a disorder characterized by decreased bone density and increased fracture risk, is more common in women, especially as they age.

Low-impact weight-bearing exercises, such as dancing or using resistance bands, serve to maintain bone density and lower the risk of osteoporosis-related fractures, promoting skeletal health and lifespan.

6. *Improved Posture and Balance:* Low-impact exercise routines need core muscle strengthening and posture improvement. Pilates and stability ball exercises, for example, focus on growing core strength, improving posture, and increasing balance, making them especially good for women who spend lengthy periods of time sitting or standing in sedentary situations.

Women who include low-impact activities into their daily routines are more likely to prioritize their health. Low-impact exercise has several benefits for women of all ages, including improved joint health and cardiovascular fitness, weight management, and stress reduction.

So, whether it's a leisurely stroll in the park, a refreshing swim, or a relaxing yoga session, every step toward embracing low-impact exercise helps to improve women's overall well-being.

Joint-Friendly Workouts

When it comes to living a healthy lifestyle, exercise is crucial for everyone, even women. However, not all women may be able to participate in high-impact activities for a variety of reasons, including joint discomfort, injury rehabilitation, and pregnancy.

Low-impact activities are a great option that gives several health advantages while placing less strain on the joints. In this thorough guide, we'll look at the numerous low-impact exercises that are appropriate for women, their advantages, and how to include them in your workout regimen.

Benefits of Low-impact Exercise for Women:

Joint Health: Low-impact workouts are soft on the joints, making them suitable for ladies suffering from arthritis or joint discomfort. They improve flexibility and mobility while not exacerbating pre-existing conditions.

Injury Prevention: High-impact activities can increase the risk of injury, particularly for women who are new to fitness or have recently recovered from an accident. Low-impact activities lower the likelihood of strains, sprains, and other injuries, allowing women to exercise safely.

Low-impact aerobic workouts such as walking, cycling, and swimming continue to give cardiovascular benefits by increasing heart health, decreasing blood pressure, and lowering the risk of heart disease.

Weight Management: Regular low-impact exercise can help you lose weight by burning calories and increasing your metabolism. When combined with a good diet, it can help women reach and maintain a healthy weight.

Stress Relief: Exercise has been shown to lower stress and increase mood by producing endorphins, the body's natural feel-good chemicals. Low-impact hobbies like yoga and tai chi integrate mindfulness and relaxation methods, which promote mental well-being.

Types of Low-impact Exercises for Women:

Walking: One of the most basic yet effective kinds of exercise, walking can be done anywhere and requires no equipment. Aim for at least 30 minutes of brisk walking most days of the week to enjoy the cardiovascular and mental health rewards.

Swimming is a low-impact activity that exercises the entire body without stressing the joints. It's especially good for ladies who have arthritis or back problems since water's buoyancy supports the body while still providing resistance.

Cycling, whether outdoor or stationary, is a low-impact workout that strengthens the legs and improves cardiovascular fitness. Change gears or riding pace to suit your fitness level.

Yoga aims to improve flexibility, strength, and balance via a sequence of postures and breathing exercises. It is appropriate for all fitness levels and may be tailored to meet specific requirements.

Pilates focuses on core strength, stability, and body awareness via regulated movements. It improves posture, muscular tone, and general body alignment while minimizing joint stress.

Adding Low-impact Exercise to Your Routine:

Start Slow: If you're new to training or returning from a hiatus, begin with shorter sessions and gradually increase the time and intensity as your fitness improves.

Mix It Up: Include a variety of low-impact workouts in your regimen to keep things fresh and minimize monotony.

To avoid overuse injuries, alternate between activities like walking, swimming, and yoga. Listen to your body.

After and during exercise, pay attention to how your body feels

If you feel any pain or discomfort, adapt the activity or attempt an alternative workout that is more pleasant for you.

Stay Consistent: Consistency is essential for seeing the effects of your training plan. Aim for at least 150 minutes of moderate-intensity activity every week, spread out across multiple days, to maintain general health and fitness.

Low-impact activities provide several benefits to women of all ages and fitness levels. Walking, swimming, yoga, and cycling can help with joint health, injury prevention, and general well-being.

Boosting Confidence and Energy

In today's world, finding time and energy to exercise can be difficult, especially for women who are juggling many commitments.
However, including low-impact workouts in your program can give a variety of advantages, including increased confidence and vitality.

Let's look at how low-impact workouts can assist women improve their physical and emotional well-being.Low-impact workouts are mild on the joints and suitable for women of all ages and fitness levels.

Walking, swimming, cycling, and yoga provide a variety of activities to meet individual interests and goals. Women who participate in these sports daily can enhance their cardiovascular health, strength, and flexibility without putting undue strain on their bodies.

One of the primary advantages of low-impact exercise is its potential to increase confidence. As women improve in their fitness journeys, they frequently feel a feeling of success and pleasure in their achievements.

 Whether it's accomplishing a difficult yoga posture, increasing walking distance, or learning a new swimming technique, each accomplishment adds to a stronger sense of self-assurance.

Regular exercise produces endorphins, the body's natural mood lifters, which can improve general mood and self-esteem.low-impact activities might assist women reduce weariness and boost energy levels.

Contrary to common assumptions, physical exercise boosts energy levels by boosting circulation and oxygenation throughout the body. Women who exercise regularly may experience less weariness and more vigor.

This increase in energy can lead to increased productivity, better attention, and a higher ability to face everyday chores with zeal and excitement.

Incorporating low-impact activities into your routine does not have to be intimidating. Starting with simple, realistic objectives and progressively increasing intensity and length can help women develop a long-term fitness regimen.

Finding pleasant and meaningful hobbies may also make being active feel like a rewarding experience rather than a duty.

To reap the full advantages of low-impact exercise, prioritize consistency and listen to your body.

Setting aside time each day for physical activity, even if it's only a brief stroll or light yoga practice, can result in significant long-term advantages in both physical and emotional well-being.

Paying attention to appropriate form and technique will help you avoid injury and have a safe and successful workout.

Low-impact exercise provides several advantages for women, including enhanced confidence and vitality.

Women who incorporate activities such as walking, swimming, cycling, and yoga into their routine can improve their physical health, emotional well-being, and sense of energy and self-assurance.

Women may improve their lives for the better by committing to low-impact exercise and maintaining a happy outlook.

Chapter 3: Strength and Tone

Strength and tone are important components of total fitness, especially for women who want to reach their health objectives with low-impact workouts. Low-impact workouts are mild on the joints but yet provide a good workout.

When it comes to strength and tone, including these exercises in your regimen may provide several benefits, such as increased muscular strength, endurance, and overall body composition.

The major purpose of low-impact workouts for women is to increase muscular strength. This is critical not just for aesthetic purposes, but also for functional fitness and injury prevention.

Women can target different muscle areas and progressively develop their strength by participating in exercises such as yoga, Pilates, or the use of resistance bands. These exercises serve to tone and shape the body while reducing the likelihood of strain or injury.

Low-impact activities are great for increasing muscular tone. While aerobic activities like jogging or cycling are primarily concerned with cardiovascular health, strength training, and toning exercises focus on specific muscle areas, assisting in the development of definition and firmness.

Squats, lunges, and planks, for example, help tone and shape the legs, glutes, and core.Low-impact workouts provide additional benefits for women besides increasing strength and tone.

They can help to improve posture and flexibility, decrease stress, and boost general well-being. Yoga, in particular, is recognized for promoting relaxation and awareness while enhancing flexibility and balance.

When introducing low-impact workouts into your regimen, it's critical to concentrate on good form and technique to optimize benefits and avoid injury.

Beginning with modest weights or resistance and progressively increasing intensity as strength grows is critical.

Incorporating a range of exercises that target different muscle groups promotes a well-rounded workout and helps to prevent overuse problems.

Consistency is also key for seeing the effects of low-impact activities. Aim for at least 30 minutes of exercise most days of the week, combining strength training with aerobic activity to create a well-rounded fitness regimen.

It's also critical to listen to your body and make any modifications, especially if you have any underlying health issues or injuries.

Women's fitness requires strength and tone, and low-impact workouts provide a safe and efficient approach to reaching these goals.

Women may improve their general health and well-being by combining workouts that focus on muscular strength and tone, while also lowering their risk of injury. With consistency and effort, anybody may obtain the required strength and tone with low-impact training.

Using Resistance Bands

Resistance bands are adaptable equipment that provide a variety of low-impact exercises appropriate for women of all fitness levels.

These elastic bands create resistance throughout the activity, allowing you to gain strength, enhance flexibility, and tone muscles without placing too much strain on your joints. Here's a complete tutorial on utilizing resistance bands for low-impact training.

Resistance bands are useful in targeting a variety of muscle areas, including the arms, legs, back, and core. Resistance bands are a gentle yet efficient way for women to tone and build their muscles without using heavy weights.

Band exercises such as bicep curls, shoulder presses, squats, and lunges can help you gain muscular definition and strength.

Flexibility and Mobility: Including resistance bands in stretching exercises helps improve flexibility and mobility. Gentle stretches using bands assist to lengthen muscles and increase range of motion, making daily tasks simpler and lowering the chance of injury. Women can use bands to stretch their hamstrings, chest, and hip flexors to enhance flexibility and avoid stiffness.

Core Stability: Strong core muscles are required to maintain appropriate posture and avoid lower back problems. Resistance bands may be used to target the core with workouts like standing twists, sitting rows, and plank variants. These exercises work the abdominal muscles, obliques, and lower back, improving core stability and balance.

Balance and Coordination: Many resistance band workouts demand balance and coordination, which improves proprioception and lowers the chance of falling, particularly as women age.

Balancing on one leg while doing bicep curls or lateral raises with bands tests stability and improves stabilizing muscles, improving general balance and coordination.

Resistance bands are useful for rehabilitation activities and injury prevention since they have a mild impact. Women recuperating from accidents or managing chronic diseases can use bands to gradually strengthen muscles and joints without increasing pre-existing problems.

Incorporating resistance band movements into regular workouts can also assist to avoid injuries by addressing muscular imbalances and maintaining good alignment.

One of the primary benefits of resistance bands is their mobility and ease. They are lightweight, small, and portable, making them ideal for home workouts, vacation, and outdoor training sessions.

Women may include resistance band workouts into their daily regimen at any time and from any location, with no equipment necessary.

Resistance bands provide women with a complete and low-impact approach to training, focusing on strength, flexibility, balance, and general wellbeing.

Women who include resistance band exercises in their fitness program can reach their health and fitness objectives while reducing the risk of injury and enjoying the convenience of at-home training.

Bodyweight Exercises

Bodyweight exercises are an excellent approach for women to maintain their fitness and health without the need for pricey gym subscriptions or equipment.

Not only are they handy, but they also provide low-impact solutions that are easy on the joints, making them appropriate for women of all ages and fitness levels.

Benefits of Bodyweight Exercise for Women:

Convenience: Bodyweight workouts may be performed anywhere and at any time, with minimum space and no equipment required. You may simply include these workouts into your daily routine whether you're at home, at work, or on the go.

Low Impact: Many bodyweight exercises are low impact, which means they are easy on the joints and lessen the chance of injury. This makes them perfect for people who have joint concerns or want a less strenuous workout.

Improves Strength and Muscle Tone: Despite the absence of weights, bodyweight workouts may successfully increase strength and muscle tone. You may tone your body by targeting different muscle groups and using your body weight as resistance.

Increases Flexibility and Balance: Many bodyweight workouts incorporate motions that enhance flexibility and balance. This is especially useful for women as they get older since it helps them avoid falls and preserve their general mobility.

Improves Cardiovascular Health: Including bodyweight workouts in your fitness program can help enhance your cardiovascular health. Exercises done in a circuit or at a high intensity can raise your heart rate and increase endurance.

Low-impact bodyweight exercises for women

Modified Push-Ups: Begin by kneeling on the floor, with your hands slightly wider than shoulder-width apart. Lower your chest to the ground while maintaining your body straight, then push back up to the starting position.

Bodyweight Squats: Position your feet hip-width apart, toes slightly turned out. Bend your knees and drop your hips to the ground, as if sitting in a chair. Keep your chest raised and your weight in your heels as you return to standing.

Lunges: Take a stride forward with one foot and lower your body until both knees are bent at a 90° angle. Keep your front knee in line with your ankle and your back knee hanging slightly above the ground. Push back to the beginning position and repeat on the opposite side.

Plank: Start in a push-up position, hands squarely beneath your shoulders. From head to heels maintain a straight line and engage your core Hold for as long as possible, striving to extend the length over time.

Incorporating these low-impact bodyweight exercises into your program can help women increase strength, flexibility, and cardiovascular health without placing too much strain on their bodies.

Remember to listen to your body, begin carefully, and gradually increase intensity as you gain strength and comfort with the exercises.

Pilates and Barre Workouts

Pilates and barre workouts are becoming increasingly popular among women looking for low-impact training programs that provide full toning, flexibility, and strength-building advantages.

These techniques emphasize regulated movements, alignment, and muscular activation, making them appropriate for people of all fitness levels, including those recuperating from injuries or trying to avoid them.

Let's look at the specifics of each and why they're great options for ladies looking for moderate yet effective exercises. Pilates promotes core strength and flexibility.

Pilates, founded by Joseph Pilates in the early twentieth century, focuses on core strength, stability, and flexibility. The exercises often include precise movements performed on a mat or with specialist equipment such as the reformer. Pilates works on deep abdominal muscles, back muscles, and pelvic floor muscles, resulting in improved posture, balance, and coordination.

Breath control is a vital Pilates technique that allows practitioners to retain focus, properly use their core muscles, and relax. Pilates provides a personalized training experience based on individual requirements and objectives, with movements spanning from beginning to intermediate levels. Barre workouts sculpt and lengthen muscles.

Barre workouts, which are inspired by ballet training, use aspects of dance, Pilates, and yoga to shape and lengthen muscles while increasing balance and flexibility. Participants use a ballet barre for support while they do short, isometric motions that target particular muscular areas such the thighs, glutes, arms, and core.

Unlike typical high-impact exercises, barre routines are mild on the joints while still offering a demanding full-body workout. Barre lessons use small weights, resistance bands, and bodyweight movements to tone muscles without adding mass, resulting in long, thin physiques.

Benefits for women:

Low Impact: Pilates and barre workouts are low-impact alternatives to high-intensity exercises, lowering the risk of injury and accommodating those with joint problems or mobility limits, making them suitable for women of all ages.

Core Strength: Strengthening the core muscles is especially advantageous for women because it promotes spinal alignment, improves posture, and lowers the chance of back discomfort, which is a significant worry

For Women who have recently given birth or who are pregnant it is particularly for them.

Flexibility: Increasing flexibility is essential for preserving joint health and avoiding stiffness, which becomes more prevalent as women age. Pilates and barre workouts use dynamic stretches and lengthening movements to increase flexibility and range of motion.

Body Confidence: Both activities encourage body awareness and mindfulness, developing a good body image and increasing self-confidence, which is beneficial to women of all shapes and sizes.

Pilates and barre workouts provide women with a comprehensive approach to training, integrating strength, flexibility, and mindfulness in moderate, low-impact programs. Whether you're a novice or an experienced fitness enthusiast, including these exercises into your regimen will enhance your physical and mental health, allowing you to look and feel your best.

Chapter 4: Aquatic Exercise

Aquatic exercise provides a complete and low-impact training choice, making it ideal for women looking for a gentle yet effective approach to increase fitness, control weight, and improve general well-being.

This type of exercise utilizes water's buoyancy and resistance to deliver a full-body workout without putting undue strain on joints and muscles. Here's a comprehensive look at the advantages and forms of aquatic workouts appropriate for women:

Benefits of Water Exercise for Women:

Low Impact: Water supports the body while decreasing joint impact, making it excellent for ladies suffering from arthritis, joint discomfort, or recuperating from an injury.

Muscle Strengthening: Water resistance works muscles without exertion, producing strength and toning throughout the body.

Cardiovascular Health: Aquatic activities can increase heart rate and enhance cardiovascular endurance, assisting with weight control and lowering the risk of heart disease.

Improved Flexibility: Water's moderate resistance promotes flexibility and range of motion, resulting in improved mobility and less stiffness.

Stress Relief: Immersion in water has a relaxing impact, lowering stress levels and encouraging relaxation, making aquatic exercise a good choice for mental health.

Types of Aquatic Exercise for Women:

Swimming laps is a full-body workout that targets muscles in the arms, legs, and core while boosting cardiovascular fitness.

Water Aerobics: These sessions usually contain a range of aerobic exercises, such as jumping jacks, leg lifts, and arm motions, which are done in shallow or deep water to increase endurance and strength.

Aquatic Yoga: Practicing yoga postures with water resistance improves balance, flexibility, and awareness while delivering a low-impact workout.

Water Walking/jogging: Walking or jogging in water exercises the lower body muscles while reducing joint stress, making it a good choice for ladies who have knee or hip problems.

Aquatic cycling involves riding a stationary cycle submerged in water, which gives a unique cardiovascular exercise while strengthening leg muscles and increasing circulation.

Water Pilates: Pilates exercises designed for the water emphasize core strength, stability, and flexibility, providing a mild yet effective technique to tone muscles and improve posture.

Including water training in your fitness program may be extremely helpful for women of all ages and fitness levels. Whether you want to lose weight, enhance your mobility, or just get a good workout, water exercise is a safe and effective choice.

Consulting with a trained water fitness teacher may help you adapt a program to your specific requirements and goals, assuring maximum benefits while lowering your risk of injury. So plunge in and discover the numerous advantages of water training for women's health and fitness!

Water's Therapeutic Benefits

Water's medicinal advantages go well beyond quenching thirst. For women looking for low-impact exercise choices, water-based activities provide a comprehensive approach to wellbeing. Here's a thorough examination of water's medicinal properties and its function in low-impact activities for women:

Joint support: The buoyancy of water lessens the impact on joints, making it a great workout setting, particularly for ladies suffering from joint discomfort or arthritis. Swimming and water aerobics allow for mild activity without putting load on fragile joints.

Immersion in water increases muscular relaxation, which relieves stress and reduces the chance of damage during activity. Water resistance progressively builds muscles, unlike the jarring impact of high-impact workouts.

Cardiovascular health: Water-based workouts, such as swimming laps or running, provide cardiovascular benefits comparable to land-based sports. Water resistance raises heart rate and promotes circulation, promoting heart health without putting the body under stress.

tension relief: The relaxing impact of water can help to relieve tension and anxiety, in addition to giving physical health advantages. Swimming's rhythmic strokes or the serene setting of a water exercise might help you relax and feel better overall.

enhanced flexibility: Water's resistance allows for a wide range of motion, which improves flexibility and mobility. Women can practice mild stretches and fluid motions in water to increase joint flexibility without risking overextension or strain.

Weight management: Water-based activities are an efficient technique to manage weight without putting undue strain on the body. Water resistance improves calorie expenditure, but the activity's low-impact nature lowers the danger of overexertion or injury.

Women recuperating from injury or surgery can benefit from water-based activities, which are both safe and effective. The buoyancy of water supports the body, allowing for regulated movement and strengthening without putting undue strain on the healing tissues.

social connection: Water-based workout programs or group activities allow women to engage and encourage one another. Connecting with individuals who have similar fitness objectives can boost motivation and pleasure of exercise.

To summarize, water's therapeutic properties make it an essential resource for women looking for low-impact workout choices. Including water-based activities in a fitness program, whether swimming laps, engaging in water aerobics, or simply taking a leisurely bath, can improve general health and well-being.

Women may attain their fitness objectives while lowering their risk of injury and increasing their enjoyment of exercise by utilizing water's healing powers.

Water Aerobics

Water aerobics, often known as aqua aerobics or water workouts, provides a delightful and efficient low-impact workout for women of all ages and fitness levels.

This type of workout uses water's inherent resistance to deliver multiple advantages while being easy on joints and muscles. Let's look at the specifics of water aerobics and its benefits for ladies looking for a balanced workout program.

1. What is water aerobics?

Water aerobics is doing various aerobic exercises in a pool, usually in shallow water. Water resistance is used to support movements including walking, running, jumping jacks, and arm workouts.

Equipment like foam dumbbells, noodles, and kickboards can also be used to intensify the workout.

2. Advantages of Water Aerobics for Women

Water buoyancy lessens the joint impact, making it perfect for ladies who have arthritis, joint discomfort, or are recuperating from an injury.

Muscle Strengthening: Water offers resistance in all directions, allowing you to tone your muscles without using heavy weights.

Cardiovascular Health: Water aerobics promote heart health and circulation, minimizing the risk of cardiovascular disease.

Improved Flexibility: Water's buoyancy helps to support and stretch muscles, increasing flexibility and range of motion.

Weight Management: Water aerobics burns calories and promotes lean muscle development, which aids with weight loss and maintenance.

Social Engagement: Group water aerobics courses promote camaraderie and encouragement, providing a supportive atmosphere for women to keep active.

3. Get Started

Consultation: Before beginning any workout regimen, speak with your healthcare professional, especially if you have any pre-existing medical concerns.

Wear a comfortable swimsuit and water shoes for traction. Pack a water bottle to remain hydrated.

Warm-up: Start with simple stretches and motions to get your muscles ready for the workout.

Start Slow: To avoid overexertion, gradually increase the intensity and length of your workouts.

Proper Form: To enhance the efficacy of each exercise, keep your posture and alignment correct.

4. Sample Water Aerobics Routine.

Warm-up: 5 minutes walking or running in place.

Cardio: 20 minutes of alternating running, jumping jacks, and cross-country skiing.

Strength Training: Perform 15 minutes of arm curls, leg lifts, and squats using foam dumbbells or resistance bands.

Cool down with five minutes of moderate stretching and deep breathing exercises.

F

Water aerobics provides a pleasant and satisfying alternative for women to be active while reducing their chance of injury.

This low-impact exercise, which uses water resistance to create a full-body workout, has various health advantages.

Whether you're a novice or a seasoned exerciser, jump into the pool and discover the exciting world of water aerobics.

Swimming for Fitness

Swimming is a wonderful type of exercise for ladies looking for a low-impact, high-intensity workout. It provides a thorough workout that activates many muscle groups while reducing joint stress, making it perfect for anyone who has joint discomfort, arthritis, or is recuperating from an accident.

Here's an in-depth look at swimming for fitness, concentrating on the advantages, methods, and advice for women.

Benefits of Swimming for Women:

Swimming, unlike high-impact workouts like jogging or weightlifting, places little strain on joints, lowering the chance of injury and offering a safe workout environment for women of all ages and fitness levels.

Swimming is a full-body workout that works for many muscle groups at the same time, such as the arms, legs, core, and back. It improves muscular strength, endurance, and flexibility, hence contributing to general fitness and body toning.

Swimming increases the heart rate, which improves cardiovascular health and lung capacity. Regular swimming helps to lower blood pressure, cholesterol levels, and the risk of heart disease and stroke.

Weight control: Swimming is a calorie-burning workout that helps with weight loss and control. Water resistance delivers a difficult workout that burns calories and promotes lean muscular growth.

Stress Relief: The regular motion of swimming, along with the pleasant sense of being in the water, promotes relaxation and lowers stress levels. It is a therapeutic exercise that relaxes the mind and improves general well-being.

Techniques For Effective Swimming:

Freestyle (Front Crawl): The most popular stroke, freestyle combines continuous arm motions with alternating kicks. It gives you great cardiovascular exercise while also improving your upper body strength.

Breaststroke: This stroke combines synchronized arm motions with a frog-like kick. Breaststroke is mild on the joints and works to tone the chest, shoulders, and thighs.

Backstroke involves swimmers lying on their backs and circularly moving their arms while kicking with their legs. Backstroke promotes posture, strengthens the back muscles, and releases stress in the neck and shoulders.

Butterfly Stroke: A more advanced stroke that combines an arm action mimicking wings fluttering with a dolphin kick. It improves core strength, flexibility, and coordination.

Tips for Women Swimming for Fitness:

Start Slowly: Begin with shorter swimming sessions and progressively increase the time and intensity as your fitness grows.

Use the Right Gear: Invest in a well-fitting swimsuit, goggles, and swim cap to guarantee comfort and efficiency in the water.

Stay Hydrated: Drink lots of water before and after swimming to keep yourself hydrated and recover lost fluids.

Practice Breathing: Focus on rhythmic breathing to increase oxygen intake and endurance when swimming.

Listen to your body. Pay attention to any discomfort or pain you experience while swimming and change your technique or intensity accordingly to avoid damage.

Swimming provides women with a varied, low-impact training alternative that improves general fitness, cardiovascular health, and stress alleviation.

Women may reap several benefits from swimming by including it in their workout program and adhering to suitable practices and advice.

Chapter 5: Walking for Wellness

Walking is one of the most basic but beneficial types of exercise, particularly for women seeking a low-impact strategy to enhance their health.

It is convenient, free, and can be adapted to individual fitness levels. Incorporating regular walking into your regimen can provide several physical and emotional health advantages.

Physical benefits of walking include its low impact on joints, making exercise suitable for ladies with joint discomfort or arthritis. Walking puts less stress on the knees, hips, and ankles than high-impact workouts like running or leaping, lowering the chance of injury.

Consistent walking promotes cardiovascular health by raising heart rate and circulation. It decreases blood pressure, lowers LDL (bad) cholesterol, and boosts overall heart function, lowering the risk of heart disease and stroke.

Walking consistently can help manage weight by burning calories and increasing metabolism. When combined with a well-balanced diet, it can help women attain and maintain a healthy weight, lowering their risk of obesity-related diseases including diabetes and certain cancers.

Walking improves muscular tone and strength, particularly targeting the lower body but also engaging the core and upper body. Over time, this can enhance muscular tone and strength, particularly in the legs, glutes, and abdominals.

Walking and other weight-bearing activities can help preserve bone density and lower the risk of osteoporosis, which is more common among women. Walking promotes bone growth, resulting in stronger, healthier bones and lowering the risk of fractures and bone-related disorders later in life.

Walking outside, particularly in natural settings such as parks or trails, can provide mental and emotional benefits, including stress reduction.

The combination of fresh air, sunlight, and physical activity reduces stress hormones like cortisol while enhancing feel-good neurotransmitters like serotonin, improving overall well-being.

Walking can improve mood by generating endorphins, which are natural mood boosters. It allows for reflection and relaxation, taking a vacation from the demands of everyday life.

Physical exercise, such as walking, improves cognitive performance by boosting blood flow and stimulating the creation of new neurons. It can boost memory, attention, and creativity, allowing women to remain cognitively sharp and attentive as they age.

Walking is a varied and accessible kind of exercise that has several benefits for women looking to enhance their health.

Whether for physical fitness, emotional well-being, or simply enjoying the great outdoors, including frequent walks into your routine may have a significant and beneficial influence on your overall health.

Walking Techniques

Walking is a great low-impact activity that has many health advantages for women of all ages. Whether you're just starting in fitness or seeking a light type of exercise, understanding good walking methods is critical for getting the most out of your workout while reducing your risk of injury.

Here's a whole reference to walking techniques designed exclusively for women:

1. Maintaining proper posture is essential for effective walking and reducing muscle and joint strain. Stand tall, with your head up, shoulders back, and abs engaged. Keep your arms loose and swing them freely when walking.

2. **Footwear:** Choosing supportive and comfortable walking shoes can avoid foot

discomfort and injuries. Look for shoes with cushioning, arch support, and a flexible sole that allows your feet to move naturally.

3. *Warm-Up:* Begin your walk with a quick warm-up to prepare your muscles and joints for exercise. To promote blood flow and flexibility, perform dynamic stretches such as leg swings, arm circles, and ankle rolls.

4. *speed:* Set a comfortable speed that allows you to walk briskly without overexertion. Aim for a speed that allows you to have a conversation without feeling out of breath. Slowly increase your pace as your fitness increases.

5. *Stride:* Take natural, flowing steps, landing heel-first and sliding easily to the toes. Avoid overstriding, since it can cause muscular tension and exhaustion. To walk efficiently, keep your stride length constant.

6. Engage core muscles by gradually bringing your navel towards your spine when walking. This helps to support your pelvis and keep it in perfect position during your stride.

7. Coordinate arm action with leg step for increased velocity and efficiency. Bend your elbows 90 degrees and swing your arms naturally in time with your opposing leg.

8. Breathing: Practice regular breathing to maintain oxygen flow to muscles and boost energy levels. Inhale deeply through your nose and exhale through your mouth in a calm and controlled way.

9. Cool Down: After your stroll, do easy stretching activities to minimize muscular pain and increase flexibility.

10. Listen to Your Body: Observe how your body feels during and after a walk. If you suffer any pain or discomfort, alter your technique or intensity as needed, and visit a healthcare practitioner if necessary.

Incorporating these walking strategies into your practice will allow you to receive the full advantages of this low-impact exercise while reducing your chance of injury. Remember to remain consistent and progressively increase the length and intensity of your walks as your fitness improves. Happy walking!

Interval Walking

Interval walking is a low-impact training plan that is extremely beneficial to women's health and fitness.

This strategy, which combines the simplicity of walking with the intensity of interval training, boosts calorie burn, improves cardiovascular health, increases endurance, and promotes general well-being while minimizing joint stress.

Interval walking consists of alternating between intervals of moderate-paced walking and brief bursts of quicker, more strenuous walking.
This change in intensity tests the body, boosts metabolic rate, and promotes fat burning. It's an excellent workout for ladies who want to reduce weight, tone muscles, and increase their fitness level without the high impact of sports like jogging or jumping.

One of the primary benefits of interval walking is its flexibility to varying fitness levels. Beginners can begin with shorter bouts of intensive walking and longer periods of moderate walking, gradually increasing the intensity and length as they gain comfort and fitness.

This versatility makes it accessible to women of various ages and fitness levels.

For women who are concerned about their joint health, interval walking offers a safer option for high-impact workouts like jogging or aerobics.

Reducing repeated stress on the joints lowers the chance of damage while still providing hard exercise. This makes it especially advantageous for people who suffer from arthritis, joint discomfort or have previously been injured.

Interval walking has considerable cardiovascular advantages. The alternating intervals of exercise and recuperation promote heart health by improving circulation, reducing blood pressure, and increasing cardiovascular endurance.

Research has shown that frequent interval training can lower the risk of heart disease, stroke, and other cardiovascular problems, making it an important part of a heart-healthy lifestyle for women.

Interval walking has been shown to improve both physical and mental well-being. Regular motion and fresh air can help relieve tension and anxiety, and boost mood. It allows women to relax, clear their brains, and connect with nature, which contributes to overall mental health.

To begin interval walking, ladies can follow this easy routine: start with a 5-minute warm-up of mild walking, then alternate between 1-2 minutes of rapid walking and 2-3 minutes of moderate walking for a total of 20-30 minutes. Finish with a 5-minute cooldown of easy walking and mild stretching to increase flexibility and reduce muscular pain.

Interval walking is a complete and successful low-impact workout choice for women looking to boost their fitness, burn calories, and improve their general well-being.

With its versatility, safety, and multiple health advantages, it's an excellent supplement to any woman's fitness program. Whether you're a novice or an experienced fitness lover, interval walking is a simple and pleasurable approach to keep active and healthy for life.

Enjoyable Walking Routes

Walking is a terrific low-impact workout that provides several health advantages to women of all ages. It not only improves cardiovascular health and helps you maintain a healthy weight, but it also boosts your mood, decreases stress, and improves your general well-being.

To make walking more pleasurable, consider taking different routes that include scenic views, tranquil environs, and fascinating locations. Here, we'll look at several extensive and detailed walking routes designed specifically for ladies seeking low-impact exercise.

1. Nature Trails: Enjoy a peaceful setting surrounded by lush foliage, animals, and fresh air. Seek out local parks, botanical gardens, or wildlife reserves with dedicated walking pathways. These routes often have modest slopes and terrain, making them excellent for low-impact training. Enjoy the views and sounds of nature while reaping physical and emotional advantages from walking.

2. *seaside Walks:* For those living near the shore, seaside walks provide a relaxing experience and spectacular ocean vistas. Choose a route along sandy beaches or cliffside trails, listening to the soothing sound of waves crashing against the coast. Coastal walks often have level terrain, which is ideal for a stroll while enjoying the sea air and soaking up vitamin D from the sun.

3. *Urban Exploration:* Discover walking paths that highlight local monuments, architecture, and cultural attractions. Walk through colorful neighborhoods, historic areas, and bustling city streets to get your daily dose of exercise. Urban walking offers route variety, guaranteeing that there is always something new to explore on each excursion.

4. *Park Circuits:* Many parks include dedicated walking or jogging circuits, including small loops and longer pathways. These circuits frequently include well-kept walkways, beautiful overlooks, and facilities like seats and drinking fountains.

Parks provide a secure and welcoming setting for women to indulge in low-impact exercise while taking in the beauty of nature.

5. *Botanical Gardens:* Enjoy a relaxing walk through brilliant blooms, exotic plants, and quiet ponds. Botanical gardens often include paved walkways with minor elevation changes, making them suitable for walkers of all fitness levels.

Take your time strolling around these wonderful gardens, admiring the many plant types and inhaling the aromatic smells.

Incorporating interesting walking routes into your routine may make exercising more fun while also improving your physical and emotional health.

Whether you like nature trails, beach walks, urban exploration, park circuits, or botanical gardens, there is a walking path to suit your interests and fitness level.

Lace-up your walking shoes, get outside, and begin on a voyage of health, enjoyment, and discovery with the power of walking.

Chapter 6: Balance and Stability

Women are increasingly discovering the need for balance and stability in their quest for overall health and wellness. These characteristics not only aid in daily tasks but also help to avoid injuries and improve general health.

Exploring unique ways to low-impact workouts designed specifically for women can bring new views and appealing alternatives to typical fitness regimens.

Unconventional, low-impact exercises for women:

Barre Fusion: This low-impact workout combines aspects of ballet, Pilates, and yoga to target muscles throughout the body. Participants use a ballet barre for support as they regulate motions and isometric holds to improve their balance, stability, and flexibility. This dynamic fusion workout pushes the body to new limits while encouraging grace and poise.

BOSU Ball Training: The BOSU (Both Sides Up) ball is a flexible instrument that adds instability to workouts, necessitating the use of stabilizing muscles.

Women may enhance their balance, proprioception, and core strength by performing many exercises on the BOSU ball, including squats, lunges, and planks. Its unique shape tests the body's balance, making it an effective yet low-impact way to improve stability.

Aerial silks, also known as aerial fabric or aerial hammocks, provide an exciting and demanding training experience. Participants are hung from the ceiling by fabric and perform dynamic exercises that involve core strength, balance, and coordination. While aerial silks may appear intimidating at first, they can be tailored to suit a variety of fitness levels, giving a fascinating and low-impact workout for ladies looking for a creative outlet.

Animal Flow is a bodyweight-based fitness regimen that focuses on fluidity, mobility, and stability. Participants imitate the motions of animals like bears, apes, and crabs, fluidly switching between positions to improve strength, flexibility, and coordination.

This primal approach to training is an enjoyable and engaging method for women to develop balance and stability while reconnecting with their natural movement patterns.

Rebounder Workouts: Rebounding, also known as mini-trampoline workouts, is a fun and effective approach to enhancing

balance, coordination, and cardiovascular fitness. Women may exercise their core muscles and lower body while bouncing on a mini-trampoline, which provides a low-impact, high-energy workout.
Rebounder routines may be tailored to include aspects of dancing, strength training, and interval training, resulting in a dynamic and exciting fitness experience.

Incorporating new low-impact activities such as Barre Fusion, BOSU ball training, aerial silks, Animal Flow, and rebounder workouts into their fitness routine may help women improve their balance, stability, and general well-being.

Women who embrace diversity in exercise techniques can discover new ways to push their bodies, broaden their skill sets, and begin on a path of self-discovery and development.

Balance Exercises

Maintaining balance is critical for our general health and well-being, particularly as we age. Balance exercises are especially important for women since they not only promote stability but also help to prevent accidents and retain independence.

Low-impact balancing exercises are a moderate but effective technique to enhance stability while avoiding unnecessary strain on joints and muscles. Here, we'll look at thorough and detailed low-impact balance exercises designed exclusively for ladies.

1. Tai Chi: This ancient Chinese martial art emphasizes slow, methodical motions and changing body weight, making it an ideal low-impact balancing exercise for women. Tai Chi increases physical strength, flexibility, and coordination while also providing relaxation and stress relief.

2. *Yoga:* Poses like Tree Pose, Warrior III, and Eagle Pose require balance and stability while simultaneously increasing flexibility and strength. Yoga, with its gentle tone and emphasis on mindfulness, is especially well-suited for women of any age.

3. *Single-Leg Stance:* Simply standing on one leg for extended periods may dramatically improve balance.

Begin by holding onto a solid surface for support if necessary, then move to independent single-leg standing. This exercise improves the muscles that surround the ankles, knees, and hips.

4. *Heel-to-Toe Walk:* In this exercise, walk in a straight line while placing the heel of one foot squarely in front of the toes of the other with each stride. It tests balance and proprioception, the body's perception of its location in space. Women can execute this workout indoors or outdoors, with a corridor or clear route for direction.

5. *Stability Ball workouts:* Using a stability ball may impart a sense of instability to typical workouts, effectively exercising core muscles and improving balance. Women may get an excellent low-impact workout with simple movements like seated or kneeling balance on the ball, ball bridges, and leg lifts.

6. *Standing Leg Lifts:* Lift one leg to the side, front, or back while keeping balance on the opposing leg.

This workout strengthens the hips, thighs, and buttocks while increasing balance and stability. Women can do standing leg lifts with or without the assistance of a chair or wall for balance.

Incorporating low-impact balancing exercises into a regular workout regimen can help women improve their stability, lower their chance of falling, and improve their overall quality of life.

Listen to your body and gradually increase the intensity and length over time. Women who prioritize balance training might gain more confidence and independence in their everyday activities.

Core Strength Training

Core strength is critical to women's overall health and fitness. A strong core helps posture and balance while also lowering the chance of injury during regular activities and exercise.

Incorporating low-impact exercises into your core strength training regimen will help women of all fitness levels develop a strong, stable core without overworking their joints and muscles.

Understand Core Strength Training:

Core strength training aims to develop the muscles in your abdominal, pelvis, lower back, and hips.

These muscles work together to support your spine, maintain good posture, and allow for mobility. Traditional core workouts such as crunches and sit-ups can be beneficial, but they may not be appropriate for everyone, particularly those with joint or back problems.

Benefits of Low-impact Exercises for Women:

Low-impact workouts are softer on the joints but yet provide an efficient workout. They lessen the chance of damage and are great for pregnant women, those recuperating from an accident, or those experiencing joint discomfort. Including low-impact exercises in your core strength training regimen will help you gain strength and stability without worsening current problems.

Effective Low-Impact Core Exercises for Women:

Plank Variations: Planks are a fundamental component of core strength training that may be changed to minimize impact. Begin with a standard forearm plank, then advance to side planks, plank rotations, and plank variants on unstable surfaces such as a stability ball.

Bird Dog: Start on your hands and knees, then extend one arm and the opposing leg while maintaining core engagement. This exercise increases balance, stability, and coordination while minimizing joint stress.

Bridge: With feet flat on the floor and knees Bent lay on the floor. Lift your hips to the ceiling while activating your glutes and core muscles. Before lowering your back down, hold for a Few seconds

Bridges help to strengthen the lower back, glutes, and hamstrings without placing strain on the spine.

Pilates movements promote core strength, flexibility, and body awareness. Many Pilates routines are low-impact and may be tailored to individual requirements. The hundred, leg circles, and single-leg stretch are all moves that efficiently target the core muscles while putting minimum effort on the joints.

Swimming: Swimming is a great low-impact workout that works the entire body, including the core. Freestyle, backstroke, and breaststroke are all excellent exercises for developing core strength while lowering joint stress.

Incorporate these low-impact core exercises into your training program to strengthen your core, increase stability, and lower your chance of injury

Get advice from a fitness expert if you have any concerns or specific health issues. With consistency and appropriate form, you can build a strong, stable core that will help you in all parts of life.

Yoga and Tai Chi

Low-impact workouts have a distinct position in the fitness world, especially for women who want to enhance their physical and mental health in a gentle but effective way.

Yoga and Tai Chi stand out among these possibilities because they are holistic activities that enhance flexibility, strength, and balance while also encouraging mindfulness and stress reduction.

Yoga, which originated in ancient India, includes some approaches that combine physical postures, breathing exercises, and meditation. Yoga provides a moderate approach to movement for women, particularly those who have joint or mobility difficulties. Poses may be changed to meet various fitness levels and physical skills, making yoga suitable for people of all ages.

In a normal yoga session, practitioners move through a sequence of asanas (poses) that stretch and strengthen muscles while encouraging relaxation and mental focus.

Downward-Facing Dog, Child's Pose, and Cat-Cow Stretch are very useful for increasing flexibility and alleviating stress in the body.

Breathing methods like deep belly breathing or alternate nostril breathing can help to quiet the mind and reduce stress, which is especially beneficial for women who have hectic schedules or suffer from anxiety.

Tai Chi, on the other hand, originated in ancient China and is commonly known as "moving meditation." This martial art emphasizes slow, methodical motions along with deep breathing and mental attention. Unlike more strenuous forms of exercise, Tai Chi is mild on the joints and muscles, making it a good choice for women wishing to enhance balance, coordination, and overall mobility without placing too much pressure on their bodies.

A typical Tai Chi practice consists of a series of flowing motions, known as forms or sequences, that are executed slowly and elegantly.

These routines encourage relaxation and awareness while also increasing physical strength and flexibility. Furthermore, Tai Chi has been demonstrated to minimize the likelihood of falls in older individuals, making it particularly advantageous for women who are concerned about keeping their balance as they age.

Both yoga and Tai Chi provide various advantages for ladies looking for low-impact workout choices. They offer an opportunity to strengthen the body, soothe the mind, and increase general well-being while avoiding injury or overexertion.

Whether performed in a group or alone, these ancient disciplines provide a comprehensive approach to fitness that can be adapted to individual requirements and interests.

Women who incorporate yoga or Tai Chi into their daily routines can achieve more physical and mental balance, as well as long-term gains in their health and vitality.

Chapter 7: Relaxation and Stress Relief

Making time to relax and reduce stress is critical to sustaining overall well-being. Balancing several duties, especially for women, may be difficult, making relaxation practices an important component of everyday routines. Low-impact workouts designed specifically for women are one excellent approach to achieve this.

Low-impact activities provide various advantages, including less stress, improved mood, greater flexibility, and improved cardiovascular health. These exercises are mild on the joints and suitable for women of all ages and fitness levels. Incorporating them into your daily routine can help reduce stress and promote relaxation.

Yoga is a popular low-impact workout that incorporates gentle movements, deep breathing, and mindfulness practices. It enhances flexibility, strength, and balance while also encouraging relaxation and stress alleviation. Women can pick from a variety of yoga styles, including Hatha, Vinyasa, and Yin, based on their tastes and fitness objectives.

Pilates is another great alternative for women looking for a low-impact workout and stress alleviation. It focuses on strengthening core muscles, improving posture, and increasing general body awareness.

Pilates movements may be adapted to meet varying fitness levels, making them appropriate for both beginners and seasoned practitioners.Walking is a simple yet effective approach for ladies to de-stress and relax.

Spending time outside, whether it's a stroll around the park or a fast walk around the block, may help clear the mind and reduce stress. Walking also allows you to connect with nature while enjoying the advantages of fresh air and sunlight.

Swimming is a low-impact sport that provides a full-body workout while being easy on your joints. Women can swim laps, take water aerobics lessons, or just float and relax in the pool.

The pleasant experience of being in the water may encourage relaxation and reduce tension, making swimming a good alternative for ladies trying to decompress.

Tai Chi is a benign martial art based on slow, flowing motions and deep breathing techniques. It enhances balance, coordination, and flexibility while encouraging relaxation and stress alleviation. Tai Chi may be performed inside or outdoors, and it is appropriate for women of all ages and fitness levels.

Incorporating low-impact activities into a woman's daily routine can have various physical and mental health advantages. Whether it's yoga, Pilates, walking, swimming, or Tai Chi, choosing activities that promote relaxation and stress alleviation is critical to overall well-being.

Making time for self-care and emphasizing relaxation can help women improve their quality of life and manage the demands of everyday living.

Meditation Techniques

Meditation is an effective technique that has been used for millennia to enhance awareness, decrease stress, and improve general well-being.

Meditation techniques vary, each having its own set of advantages and ways to quiet the mind and connect with the present moment. Below, we look at some of the most successful and widely utilized meditation techniques:

Mindfulness meditation is a practice in which you focus on the present moment without judgment. Practitioners frequently focus on their breath, physical sensations, or external stimuli like noises or images. The idea is to recognize and acknowledge thoughts and feelings as they come, rather than becoming caught up in them.

Transcendental Meditation (TM) is a practice in which practitioners silently repeat a mantra, a word or sound to attain deep relaxation and increased awareness. The mantra serves as a focal point, helping the mind to relax and become more clear.

Loving-Kindness Meditation (Metta) entails fostering sentiments of love, compassion, and goodwill for oneself and others. Practitioners frequently repeat affirmations or words like "May I be happy, healthy, and at peace," extending similar wishes to loved ones, acquaintances, and eventually all beings.

Body Scan Meditation: This technique involves carefully scanning one's body, paying attention to any sensations or tensions that arise.

By bringing awareness to each aspect of the body, practitioners can relieve physical and mental stress, fostering relaxation and a sense of completeness.

Walking meditation blends physical exercise and mindfulness practice. Practitioners concentrate on the sensation of each stride, the rhythm of their breathing, and the surroundings. This technique is especially useful for people who struggle with sitting meditation or prefer a more active approach.

Visualization meditation is the practice of mentally envisioning a tranquil setting or desired goal. Practitioners utilize their imagination to generate vivid pictures that engage all of their senses, inducing emotions of relaxation and optimism. Visualization can assist to decrease stress, boost motivation, and improve general well-being.

Breath Awareness Meditation: This approach includes merely watching the breath without attempting to control it.

Practitioners concentrate on the feeling of the breath as it enters and exits the body, enabling it to ground their attention in the present now.

Incorporating meditation into your daily practice may have a significant impact on your mental and physical health. Whether you want to relieve stress, find emotional equilibrium, or grow spiritually, there is a meditation technique for you.

By making time for practice regularly and being open to the process, you may create more mindfulness, resilience, and inner peace in your life.

Relaxation Practices

Making time to rest and unwind is critical to sustaining overall well-being. Incorporating relaxation methods into your routine, particularly low-impact activities, may dramatically enhance both your physical and mental health.

These exercises are mild on the body yet provide multiple advantages, making them appropriate for people of all ages and fitness levels.

Yoga is a popular relaxing exercise. Yoga combines gentle movements, regulated breathing, and mindfulness methods to help you relax and reduce stress. Child's Pose, Cat-Cow Stretch, and Corpse Pose all assist to relax the muscles, increase flexibility, and soothe the mind. Yoga also improves sleep quality, temperament, and general energy levels.

Tai Chi is another low-impact workout that involves slow, deliberate motions and deep breathing. Tai Chi, derived from traditional Chinese martial arts, stresses balance, coordination, and relaxation.

Regular Tai Chi practice can help with posture, joint pain relief, and cognitive function. Its contemplative feature improves brain clarity and emotional well-being.

Swimming and aqua aerobics are wonderful relaxing exercises for folks who enjoy water. Water's buoyancy relieves tension on joints and muscles, making it an excellent solution for people who have mobility concerns or chronic discomfort.

Swimming exercises the entire body, improving cardiovascular health, muscle strength, and endurance. Furthermore, the regular rhythms and soothing nature of water have a relaxing impact on the mind, which helps to reduce tension and anxiety.

Walking is a simple yet effective low-impact workout that you can do practically any place. Walking, whether it's a stroll in the park or a quick walk around the block, helps you connect with nature, clear your thoughts, and boost your mood.

According to studies, daily walking can lower blood pressure, reduce the risk of chronic illnesses, and improve mental health. To increase the relaxing effects, consider combining mindfulness practices like concentrating on your breath or analyzing your surroundings while walking.

In addition to these specific exercises, mindfulness meditation can be used as a single relaxing technique or in conjunction with other low-impact activities. Mindfulness meditation is the practice of paying attention to the present moment without judgment, which can help decrease stress, increase self-awareness, and foster a sense of peace. You may strengthen your mind-body connection and increase the effects of relaxation by practicing mindfulness while exercising.

Incorporating relaxation techniques into your workout regimen is critical for keeping a good balance in life. Low-impact workouts like yoga, Tai Chi, swimming, strolling, and mindfulness meditation provide significant physical and mental health advantages while also allowing you to relax and de-stress.

Whether you have a hectic schedule or suffer from mobility, there are several solutions available to help you relax, revitalize, and enhance your overall well-being.

Deep Breathing Exercises

Deep breathing exercises are a great low-impact practice for ladies who want to enhance their general health and well-being.

These exercises have several advantages, including stress relief, increased lung capacity, greater attention, and relaxation.

Deep breathing exercises, whether incorporated into a routine or used during stressful times, are a simple yet effective technique for reaching balance and peace in both body and mind.

To begin a deep breathing exercise, choose a comfortable, peaceful place to sit or lie down without distractions. Close your eyes and take a moment to concentrate on your breathing. Begin by breathing deeply through your nose, allowing your belly to fully expand while you fill your lungs with air. Hold this breath for a few seconds before gently and thoroughly exhaling through your lips, releasing any tension or stress with each outer breath. Repeat for several minutes, allowing each inhale and exhalation to deepen and relax.

Diaphragmatic breathing, or belly breathing, is a common deep breathing method. This approach promotes deep, regular breathing by focusing on the movement of the diaphragm, a big muscle positioned underneath the lungs.

To practice diaphragmatic breathing, place one hand on your belly and the other on your chest. As you inhale deeply, feel your belly lift and expand while your chest remains relatively motionless.

Exhale gently, allowing your abdomen to slide back into your spine. This approach promotes a sensation of peace and relaxation, reduces muscular tension, and thoroughly oxygenates the body.

The 4-7-8 method is also an excellent deep breathing practice. To practice this method, inhale deeply with your nose for four seconds, then hold your breath for seven seconds before slowly exhaling through your mouth for eight seconds.

Repeat this cycle numerous times, progressively increasing the length of each breath as you get more familiar with the method. The 4-7-8 method is especially good in inducing a state of relaxation and may be used to manage anxiety or tension.

Including deep breathing exercises in your daily routine can have a big impact on women's health and well-being. These exercises not only assist to relax and reduce tension, but they also improve lung function, boost oxygen flow to the brain and muscles, and improve mental clarity and attention.

Deep breathing exercises, whether done alone or in conjunction with other types of exercise like yoga or tai chi, are a simple yet effective technique for women to improve their overall health and energy.

CONCLUSION

Embracing low-impact exercise for women has several benefits that go beyond physical health. Throughout this research, we've looked at the numerous factors that make low-impact exercise a feasible and beneficial option for women of all ages and fitness levels.

Low-impact exercise offers a comprehensive answer for women seeking long-term fitness regimens, from its mild yet effective approach to boosting cardiovascular health to its function in increasing mental well-being.

One of the most important lessons is the inclusiveness of low-impact activities, which cater to people with a variety of needs and abilities. Whether pregnant women looking for safe forms of physical activity, seniors looking to maintain mobility, or people recovering from injuries, the versatility of low-impact exercises means that everyone can participate in regular fitness activities without risking exacerbating existing conditions or causing harm.

The accessibility of low-impact activities makes them ideal for ladies with hectic schedules. The ability to participate in activities such as swimming, cycling, walking, or yoga helps women to easily integrate exercise into their daily routines, boosting consistency and long-term commitment.

This not only promotes physical health, but also instills a sense of confidence and self-efficacy in women as they see actual increases in their strength, endurance, and general well-being over time.

Low-impact exercise also has significant psychological advantages that cannot be understated. Women who practice tai chi or Pilates might feel lower stress, greater mood, and increased body awareness.

This mind-body link promotes a good relationship with exercise, moving the emphasis away from reaching aesthetic objectives and toward embracing movement as a source of self-care and expression.

The risk of damage associated with high-impact activities is greatly decreased by low-impact alternatives, allowing women to prioritize safety while maintaining effectiveness. By focusing on good form,

THANK YOU PAGE

Thank you for selecting this book. Your support is really appreciated. Similarly, I am grateful for the purchase of this book.

Your input is valuable; please share your ideas in a review. It serves as a reference for future improvements. Enjoy reading and utilizing it!

workout planner to help keep record of progress

Weekly
Workout Planner

Week : ______________

Month: ______________

Sunday

Monday

Tuesday

Goals

Goals

Goals

Wednesday

Thursday

Friday

Goals

Goals

Goals

Saturday

Goals

Mood

Motivation ________________________

For women

Weekly
Workout Planner

Week: ________

Month: ________

Sunday

Monday

Tuesday

Goals

Goals

Goals

Wednesday

Thursday

Friday

Goals

Goals

Goals

Saturday

Goals

Mood

Motivation ________

For women

Weekly
Workout Planner

Week: _______________

Month: _______________

Sunday	Monday	Tuesday
Goals	Goals	Goals

Wednesday	Thursday	Friday
Goals	Goals	Goals

Saturday

Goals	Mood

Motivation _______________

For women

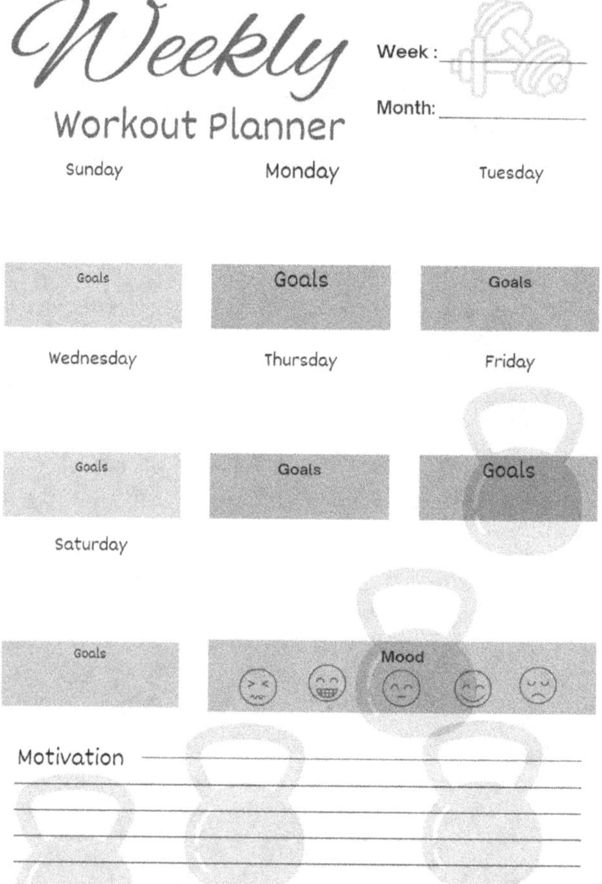

Weekly
Workout Planner
Week :
Month:
Sunday
Monday
Tuesday
Goals
Goals
Goals
Wednesday
Thursday
Friday
Goals
Goals
Goals
Saturday
Goals
Mood
Motivation
For women

Weekly
Workout Planner

Week : _______________

Month: _______________

Sunday

Monday

Tuesday

Goals

Goals

Goals

Wednesday

Thursday

Friday

Goals

Goals

Goals

Saturday

Goals

Mood

Motivation _______________________________
____
____
____
____

For women

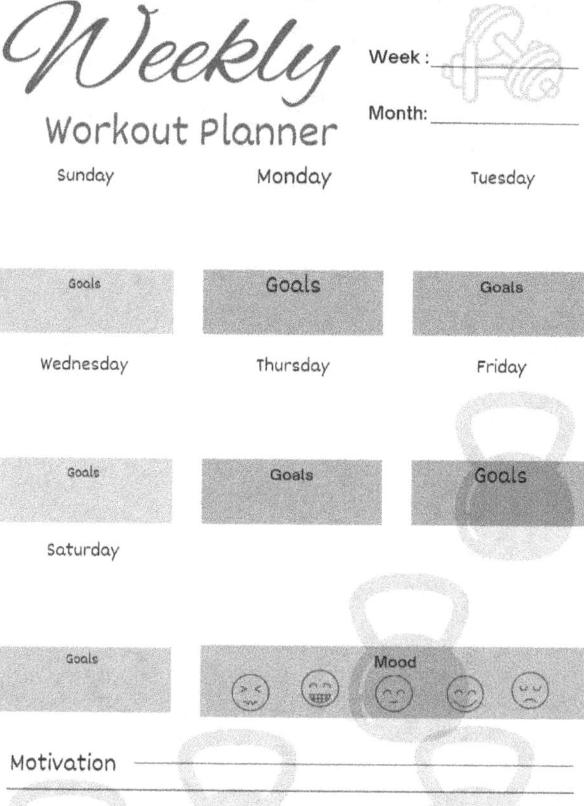

Weekly
Workout Planner
Week :
Month:
Sunday
Monday
Tuesday
Goals
Goals
Goals
Wednesday
Thursday
Friday
Goals
Goals
Goals
Saturday
Goals
Mood
Motivation
For women

Weekly

Workout Planner

Week : _______________

Month: _______________

Sunday

Monday

Tuesday

Goals

Goals

Goals

Wednesday

Thursday

Friday

Goals

Goals

Goals

Saturday

Goals

Mood

Motivation _______________

____

____

____

For women

Weekly
Workout Planner

Week: _______________

Month: _______________

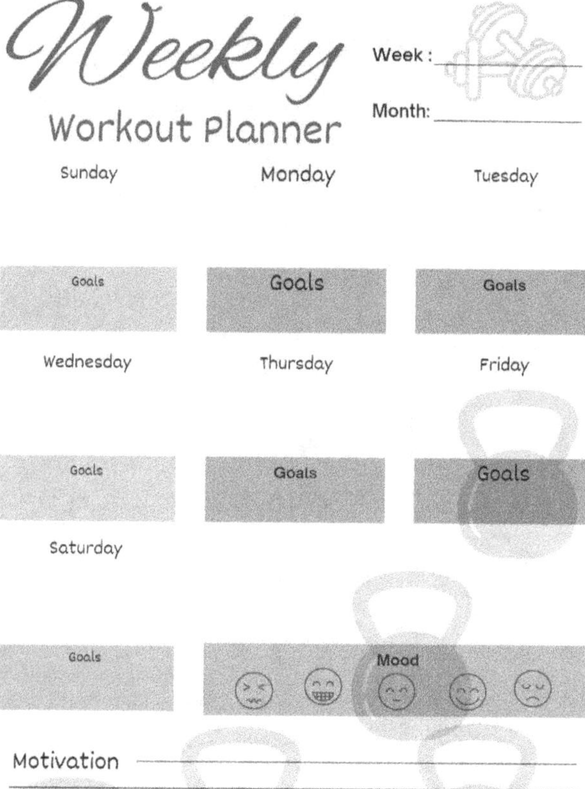

Sunday

Monday

Tuesday

Goals

Goals

Goals

Wednesday

Thursday

Friday

Goals

Goals

Goals

Saturday

Goals

Mood

Motivation _______________

For women

Weekly

Workout Planner

Week : _______________

Month: _______________

Sunday

Monday

Tuesday

Goals

Goals

Goals

Wednesday

Thursday

Friday

Goals

Goals

Goals

Saturday

Goals

Mood

Motivation _______________

For women

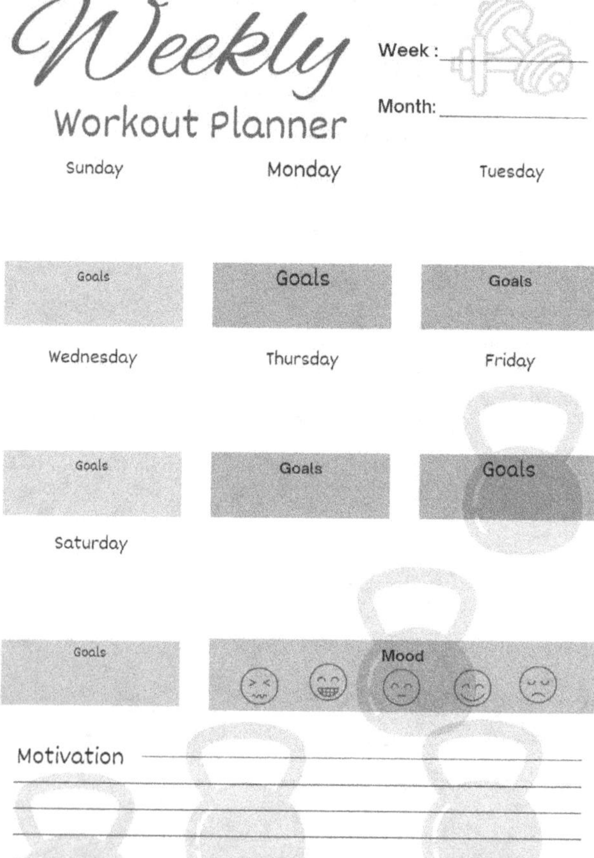

Weekly
Workout Planner
Week :
Month:
Sunday
Monday
Tuesday
Goals
Goals
Goals
Wednesday
Thursday
Friday
Goals
Goals
Goals
Saturday
Goals
Mood
Motivation
For women

Weekly
Workout Planner

Week: ______________

Month: ______________

Sunday	Monday	Tuesday
Goals	Goals	Goals

Wednesday	Thursday	Friday
Goals	Goals	Goals

Saturday		
Goals	Mood	

Motivation ________________
____
____
____
____

For women

Weekly Workout Planner

Week : __________
Month: __________

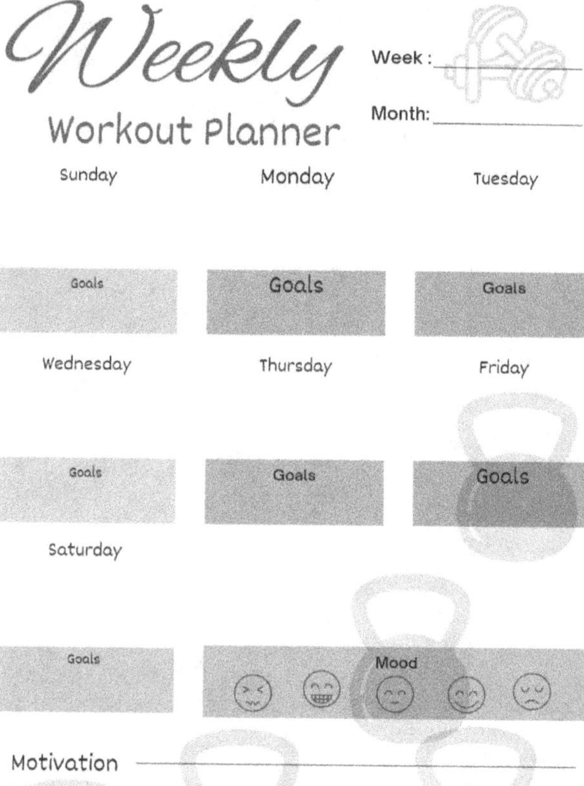

Sunday	Monday	Tuesday
Goals	Goals	Goals

Wednesday	Thursday	Friday
Goals	Goals	Goals

Saturday		
Goals	Goals	Mood

Motivation _______________________

For women

Weekly
Workout Planner

Week : _______________

Month: _______________

Sunday

Monday

Tuesday

Goals

Goals

Goals

Wednesday

Thursday

Friday

Goals

Goals

Goals

Saturday

Goals

Mood

Motivation _______________
____
____
____
____

For women

Weekly
Workout Planner

Week : ________

Month: ________

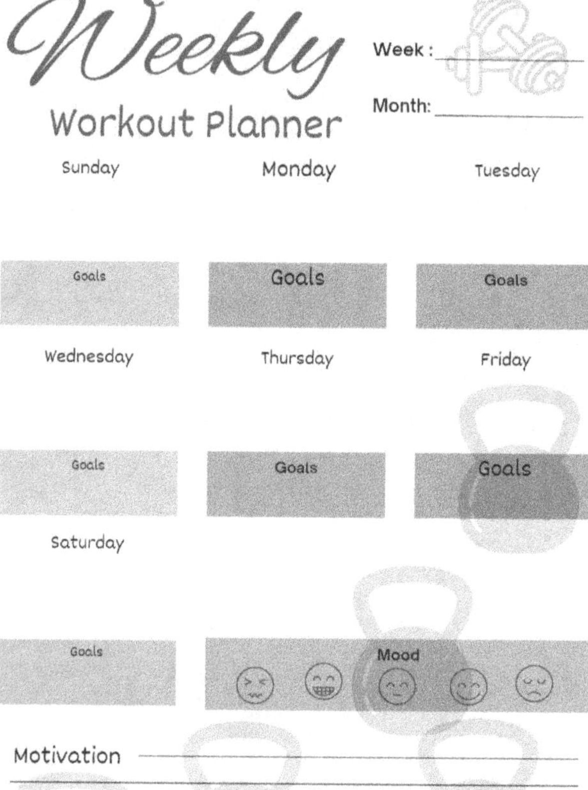

Sunday	Monday	Tuesday
Goals	Goals	Goals

Wednesday	Thursday	Friday
Goals	Goals	Goals

Saturday		
Goals		Mood

Motivation ________

For women

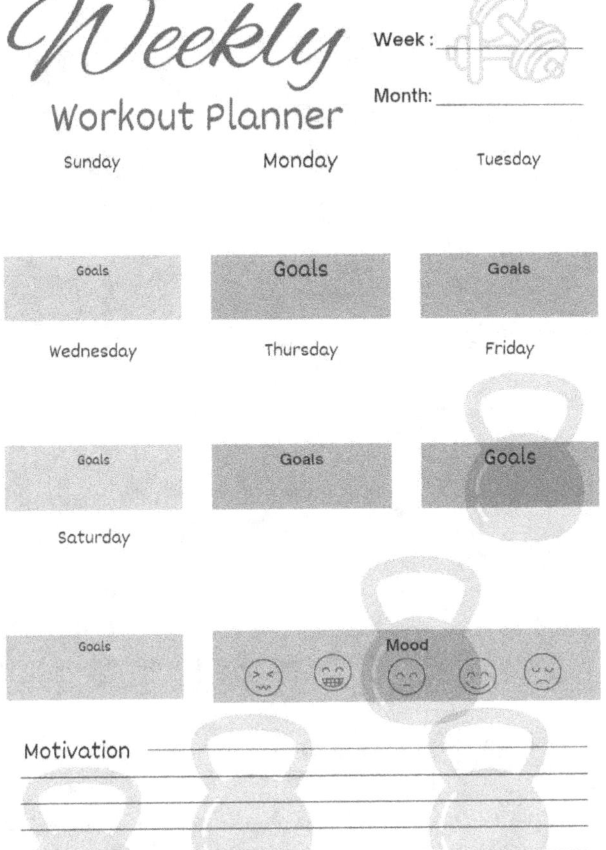

Weekly
Workout Planner
Week :
Month:
Sunday
Monday
Tuesday
Goals
Goals
Goals
Wednesday
Thursday
Friday
Goals
Goals
Goals
Saturday
Goals
Mood
Motivation
For women

Weekly
Workout Planner

Week : ________
Month: ________

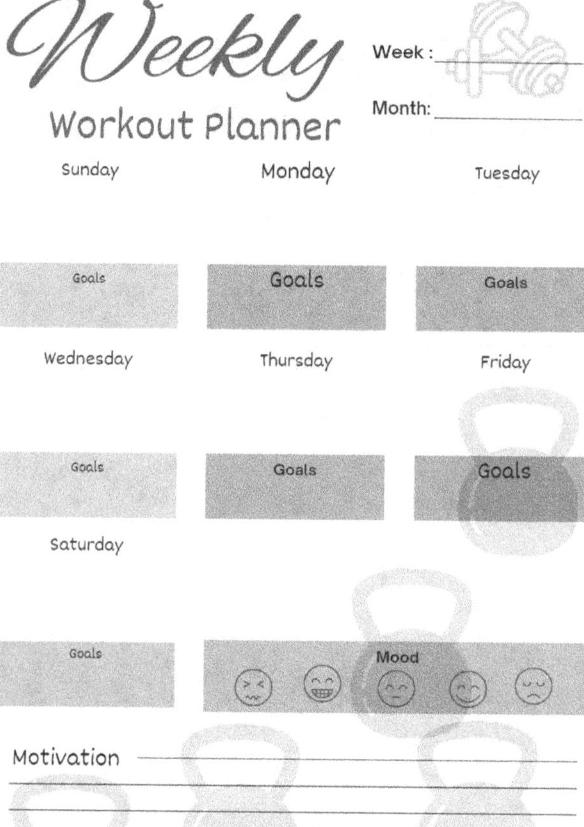

Sunday	Monday	Tuesday
Goals	Goals	Goals

Wednesday	Thursday	Friday
Goals	Goals	Goals

Saturday		
Goals	Mood	

Motivation ________________________
____
____
____
____

For women

Weekly
Workout Planner

Week : ________________

Month: ________________

Sunday

Monday

Tuesday

Goals

Goals

Goals

Wednesday

Thursday

Friday

Goals

Goals

Goals

Saturday

Goals

Mood

Motivation ________________
____
____
____
____

For women

Weekly
Workout Planner

Week : _______________

Month: _______________

Sunday	Monday	Tuesday
Goals	Goals	Goals

Wednesday	Thursday	Friday
Goals	Goals	Goals

Saturday		
Goals	Mood	

Motivation _______________

For women

Weekly
Workout Planner

Week : _______________

Month: _______________

Sunday

Monday

Tuesday

Goals

Goals

Goals

Wednesday

Thursday

Friday

Goals

Goals

Goals

Saturday

Goals

Mood

Motivation _______________
____
____
____
____

For women

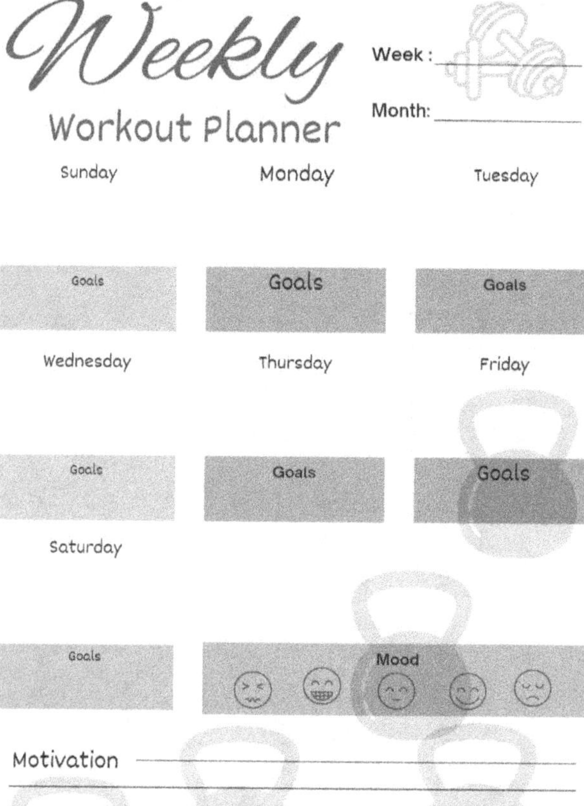

Weekly
Workout Planner

Week: _______________

Month: _______________

Sunday

Monday

Tuesday

Goals

Goals

Goals

Wednesday

Thursday

Friday

Goals

Goals

Goals

Saturday

Goals

Mood

Motivation _______________
____
____
____
____

For women

Weekly
Workout Planner

Week : ______________

Month: ______________

Sunday	Monday	Tuesday
Goals	Goals	Goals

Wednesday	Thursday	Friday
Goals	Goals	Goals

Saturday		
Goals	Mood	

Motivation ________________________________

____

____

____

For women

Weekly
Workout Planner

Week : _______________

Month: _______________

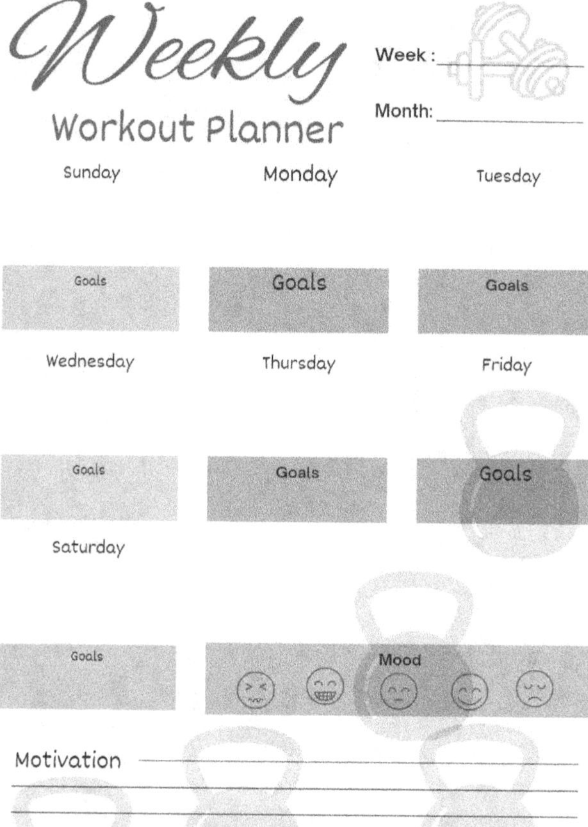

Sunday	Monday	Tuesday
Goals	Goals	Goals
Wednesday	Thursday	Friday
Goals	Goals	Goals
Saturday		
Goals	Mood	

Motivation _______________

For women

Weekly
Workout Planner
Week :
Month:
Sunday
Monday
Tuesday
Goals
Goals
Goals
Wednesday
Thursday
Friday
Goals
Goals
Goals
Saturday
Goals
Mood
Motivation
For women

Weekly
Workout Planner

Week: _____________

Month: _____________

Sunday	Monday	Tuesday
Goals	Goals	Goals

Wednesday	Thursday	Friday
Goals	Goals	Goals

Saturday		
Goals	Mood	

Motivation _________________

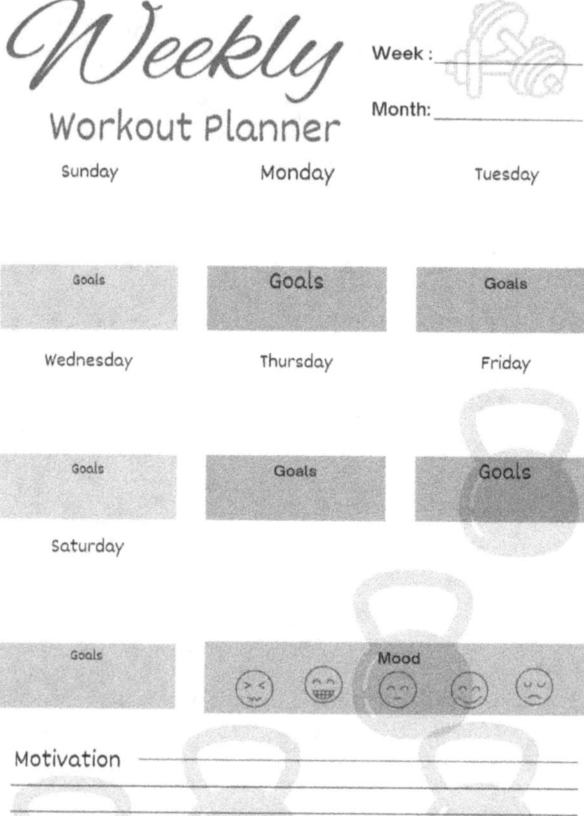

Weekly
Workout Planner

Week : _______________

Month: _______________

Sunday

Monday

Tuesday

Goals

Goals

Goals

Wednesday

Thursday

Friday

Goals

Goals

Goals

Saturday

Goals

Mood

Motivation _______________

For women

Weekly
Workout Planner

Week : _______________

Month: _______________

Sunday	Monday	Tuesday
Goals	Goals	Goals

Wednesday	Thursday	Friday
Goals	Goals	Goals

Saturday

Goals

Mood

Motivation _______________

For women

Weekly
Workout Planner

Week : ___________

Month: ___________

Sunday   Monday   Tuesday

Goals   Goals   Goals

Wednesday   Thursday   Friday

Goals   Goals   Goals

Saturday

Goals   Mood

Motivation __________________

For women

Weekly
Workout Planner

Week : _______________

Month: _______________

Sunday

Monday

Tuesday

Goals

Goals

Goals

Wednesday

Thursday

Friday

Goals

Goals

Goals

Saturday

Goals

Mood

Motivation ________________________
____
____
____
____

For women

Weekly
Workout Planner

Week : _______________

Month: _______________

Sunday

Monday

Tuesday

Goals

Goals

Goals

Wednesday

Thursday

Friday

Goals

Goals

Goals

Saturday

Goals

Mood

Motivation _______________
____
____
____
____

For women

Weekly
Workout Planner

Week : _______________

Month: _______________

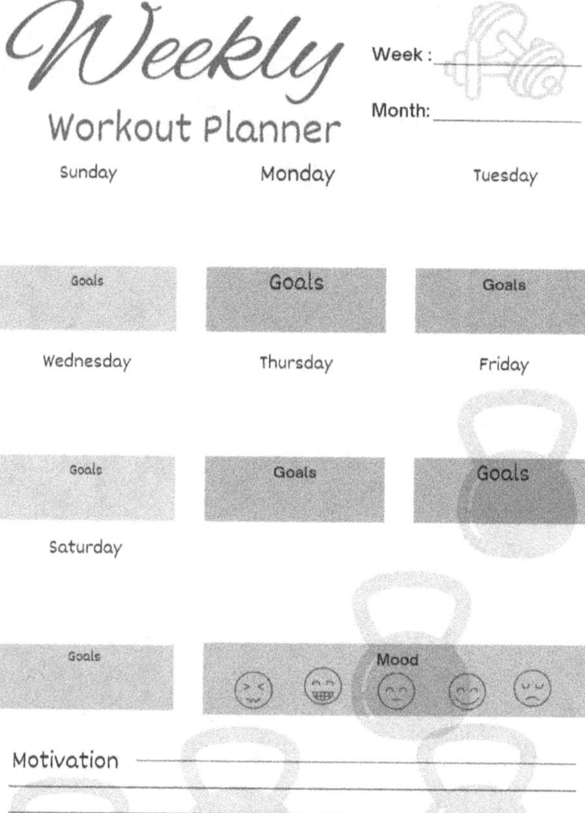

Weekly
Workout Planner

Week : _______________

Month: _______________

Sunday

Monday

Tuesday

Goals

Goals

Goals

Wednesday

Thursday

Friday

Goals

Goals

Goals

Saturday

Goals

Mood

Motivation _______________

For women

Weekly
Workout Planner

Week : ___________

Month: ___________

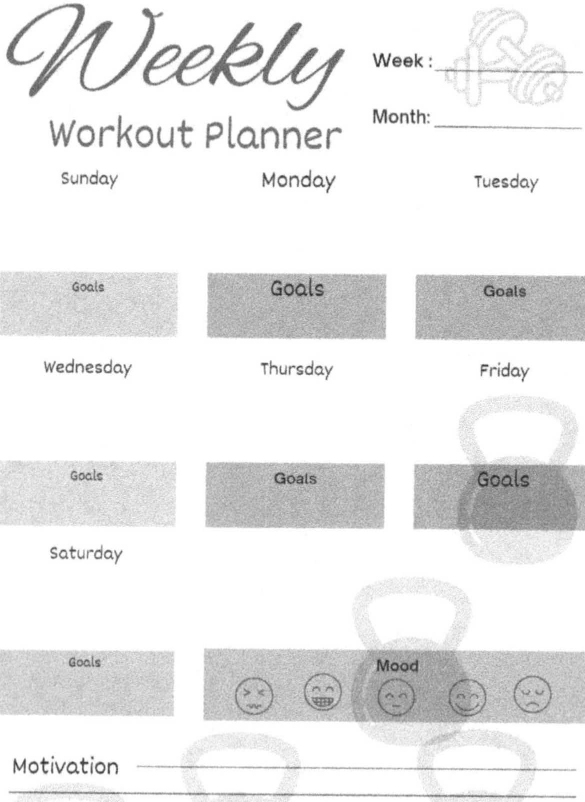

Sunday

Monday

Tuesday

Goals

Goals

Goals

Wednesday

Thursday

Friday

Goals

Goals

Goals

Saturday

Goals

Mood

Motivation

For women

Weekly
Workout Planner

Week : _______________

Month: _______________

Sunday

Monday

Tuesday

Goals

Goals

Goals

Wednesday

Thursday

Friday

Goals

Goals

Goals

Saturday

Goals

Mood

Motivation _______________
____
____
____
____

For women

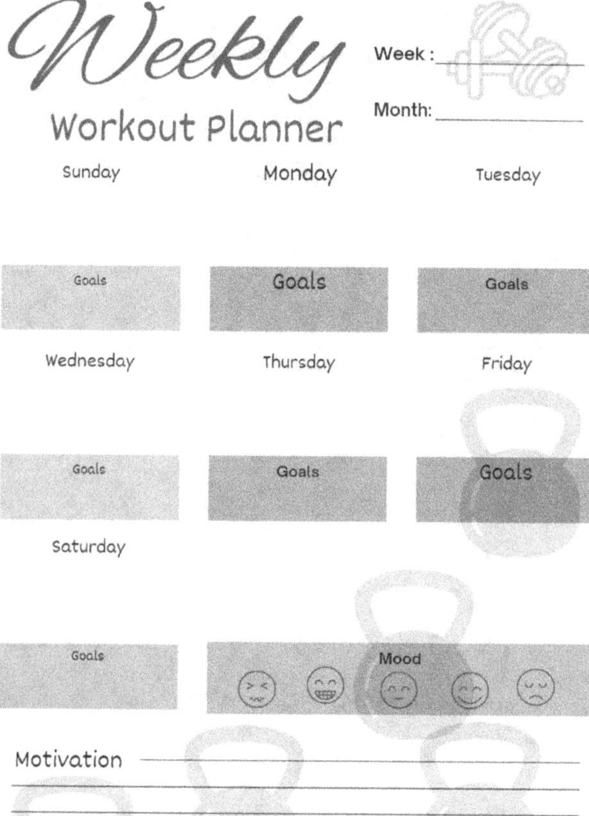

Weekly
Workout Planner

Week : _______________

Month: _______________

Sunday	Monday	Tuesday
Goals	Goals	Goals

Wednesday	Thursday	Friday
Goals	Goals	Goals

Saturday

Goals

Mood

Motivation _______________

For women

Weekly
Workout Planner

Week : _______________

Month: _______________

Sunday

Monday

Tuesday

Goals

Goals

Goals

Wednesday

Thursday

Friday

Goals

Goals

Goals

Saturday

Goals

Mood

Motivation _______________
____
____
____

For women

Weekly

Workout Planner

Week : _______________

Month: _______________

Sunday

Monday

Tuesday

Goals

Goals

Goals

Wednesday

Thursday

Friday

Goals

Goals

Goals

Saturday

Goals

Mood

Motivation _______________
____
____
____
____
____

For women

Weekly
Workout Planner

Week : ___________

Month: ___________

Sunday · Monday · Tuesday

Goals

Goals

Goals

Wednesday · Thursday · Friday

Goals

Goals

Goals

Saturday

Goals

Mood

Motivation ________________________
____
____
____

For women

Weekly Workout Planner

Week : _______________

Month: _______________

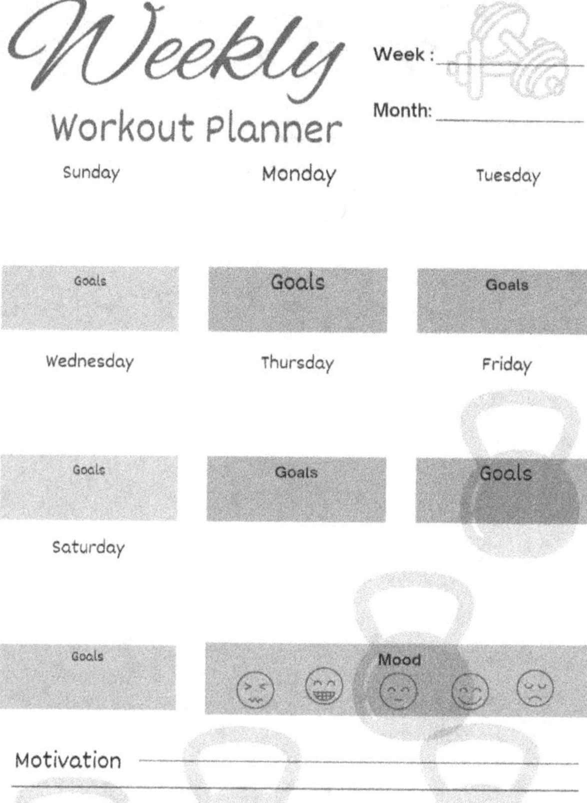

Sunday	Monday	Tuesday
Goals	Goals	Goals

Wednesday	Thursday	Friday
Goals	Goals	Goals

Saturday	Mood
Goals	

Motivation _______________

For women

Weekly
Workout Planner

Week : ___________

Month: ___________

Sunday

Monday

Tuesday

Goals

Goals

Goals

Wednesday

Thursday

Friday

Goals

Goals

Goals

Saturday

Goals

Mood

Motivation ___________________________

For women

Weekly
Workout Planner

Week : ___________

Month: ___________

| Sunday | Monday | Tuesday |

Goals · Goals · Goals

| Wednesday | Thursday | Friday |

Goals · Goals · Goals

| Saturday |

Goals

Mood

Motivation ________________________________

For women

Weekly
Workout Planner

Week: _______________

Month: _______________

Sunday

Monday

Tuesday

Goals

Goals

Goals

Wednesday

Thursday

Friday

Goals

Goals

Goals

Saturday

Goals

Mood

Motivation _______________
____
____
____
____
____

For women

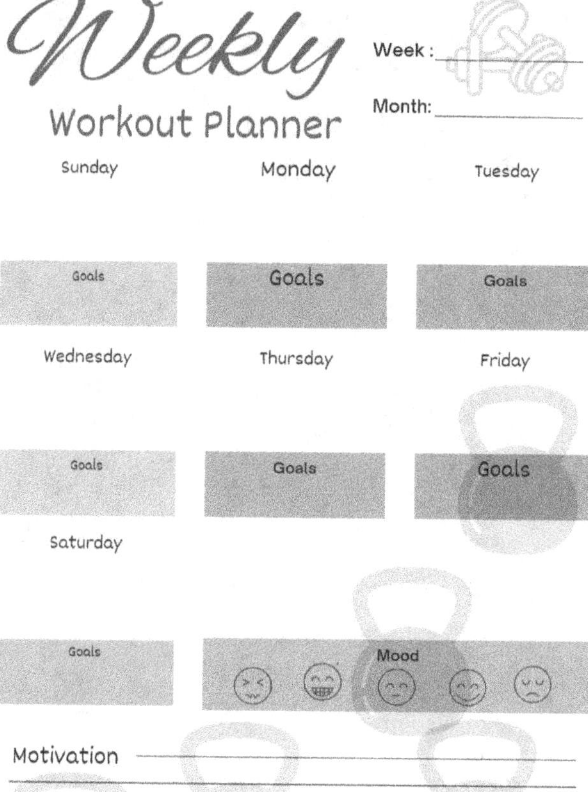

Weekly
Workout Planner

Week : _______________

Month: _______________

Sunday

Monday

Tuesday

Goals

Goals

Goals

Wednesday

Thursday

Friday

Goals

Goals

Goals

Saturday

Goals

Mood

Motivation _______________

For women

Weekly
Workout Planner

Week : _______________

Month: _______________

Sunday

Monday

Tuesday

Goals

Goals

Goals

Wednesday

Thursday

Friday

Goals

Goals

Goals

Saturday

Goals

Mood

Motivation _______________

For women

Weekly
Workout Planner

Week: _______________

Month: _______________

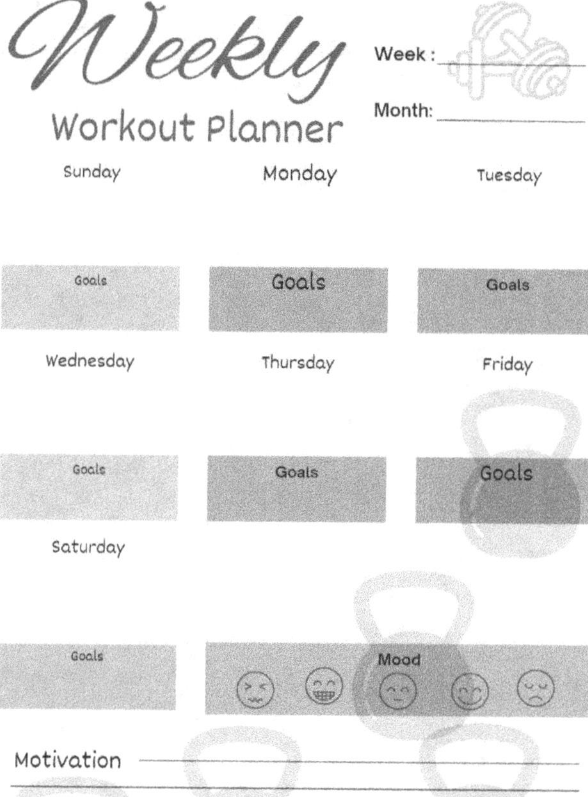

Sunday	Monday	Tuesday
Goals	Goals	Goals

Wednesday	Thursday	Friday
Goals	Goals	Goals

Saturday	Mood
Goals	

Motivation ________________________

____

____

____

____

For women

Weekly
Workout Planner

Week : ________________

Month: ________________

Sunday

Monday

Tuesday

Goals

Goals

Goals

Wednesday

Thursday

Friday

Goals

Goals

Goals

Saturday

Goals

Mood

Motivation ________________

For women

Weekly
Workout Planner

Week : _______________

Month: _______________

Sunday   Monday   Tuesday

Goals   Goals   Goals

Wednesday   Thursday   Friday

Goals   Goals   Goals

Saturday

Goals   Mood

Motivation _______________________________
____
____
____
____

For women

Weekly
Workout Planner

Week : _______________

Month: _______________

Sunday

Monday

Tuesday

Goals

Goals

Goals

Wednesday

Thursday

Friday

Goals

Goals

Goals

Saturday

Goals

Mood

Motivation ___________________
____
____
____
____

For women

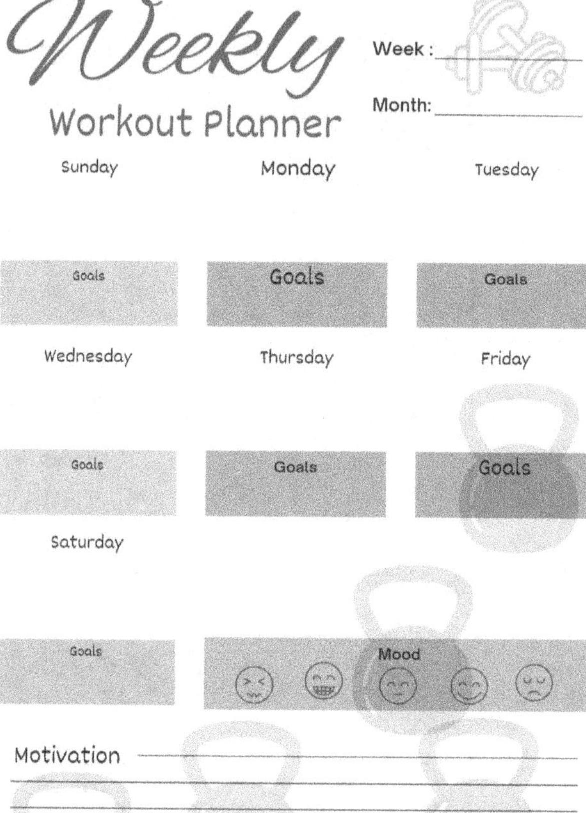

Weekly
Workout Planner
Week :
Month:
Sunday
Monday
Tuesday
Goals
Goals
Goals
Wednesday
Thursday
Friday
Goals
Goals
Goals
Saturday
Goals
Mood
Motivation
For women

Weekly
Workout Planner

Week : ___________

Month: ___________

Sunday

Monday

Tuesday

Goals

Goals

Goals

Wednesday

Thursday

Friday

Goals

Goals

Goals

Saturday

Goals

Mood

Motivation ___________________________

For women

Weekly
Workout Planner

Week : ______________

Month: ______________

Sunday	Monday	Tuesday
Goals	Goals	Goals

Wednesday	Thursday	Friday
Goals	Goals	Goals

Saturday		
Goals	Mood	

Motivation ________________________

____

____

____

____

For women

Weekly
Workout Planner

Week : __________
Month: __________

Sunday

Monday

Tuesday

Goals

Goals

Goals

Wednesday

Thursday

Friday

Goals

Goals

Goals

Saturday

Goals

Mood

Motivation ________________________________

For women

186

Weekly
Workout Planner

Week : ___________

Month: ___________

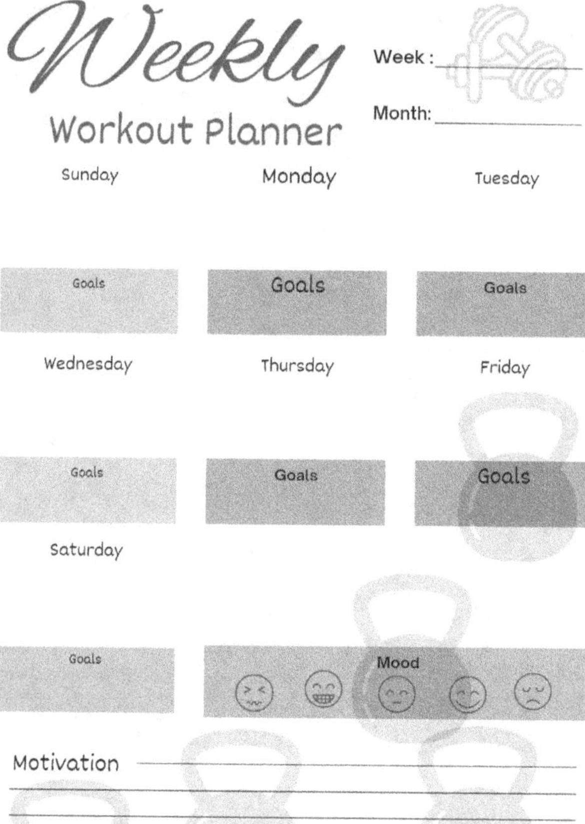

Sunday	Monday	Tuesday
Goals	Goals	Goals

Wednesday	Thursday	Friday
Goals	Goals	Goals

Saturday		
Goals	Mood	

Motivation ___________

____

____

____

____

For women

Weekly
Workout Planner

Week : ___________

Month: ___________

Sunday

Monday

Tuesday

Goals

Goals

Goals

Wednesday

Thursday

Friday

Goals

Goals

Goals

Saturday

Goals

Mood

Motivation __________________________
____
____
____
____

For women

Weekly
Workout Planner

Week: _______

Month: _______

Sunday

Monday

Tuesday

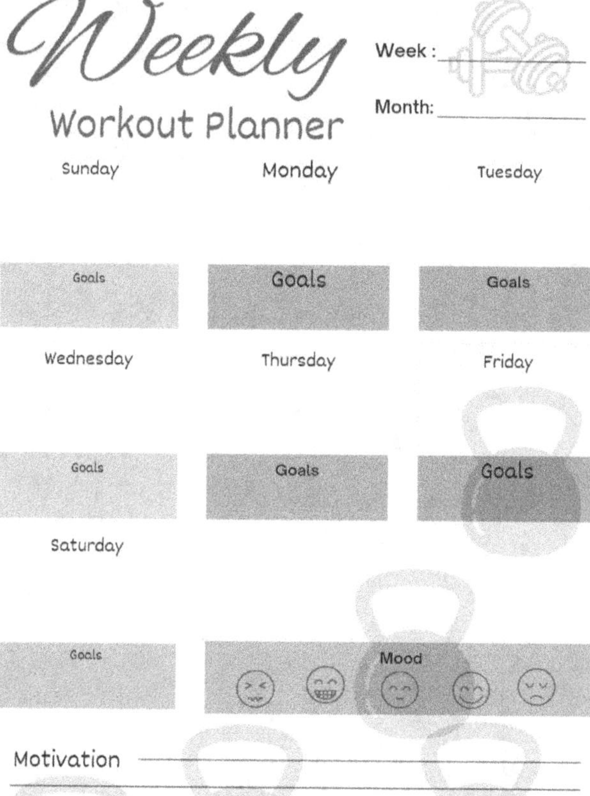

Goals

Goals

Goals

Wednesday

Thursday

Friday

Goals

Goals

Goals

Saturday

Goals

Mood

Motivation _______________________________

____

____

____

____

For women

www.ingramcontent.com/pod-product-compliance
Lightning Source LLC
Chambersburg PA
CBHW050810260726
48660CB00004B/1344